D0758150

LEGACY

LEGACY

A GENETIC HISTORY OF THE JEWISH PEOPLE

HARRY OSTRER

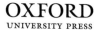
OXFORD
UNIVERSITY PRESS

OXFORD

UNIVERSITY PRESS

Oxford University Press, Inc., publishes works that further
Oxford University's objective of excellence
in research, scholarship, and education.

Oxford   New York
Auckland   Cape Town   Dar es Salaam   Hong Kong   Karachi
Kuala Lumpur   Madrid   Melbourne   Mexico City   Nairobi
New Delhi   Shanghai   Taipei   Toronto

With offices in
Argentina   Austria   Brazil   Chile   Czech Republic   France   Greece
Guatemala   Hungary   Italy   Japan   Poland   Portugal   Singapore
South Korea   Switzerland   Thailand   Turkey   Ukraine   Vietnam

Copyright © 2012 by Oxford University Press, Inc.

Published by Oxford University Press, Inc.
198 Madison Avenue, New York, New York 10016
www.oup.com

Oxford is a registered trademark of Oxford University Press

Library of Congress Cataloging-in-Publication Data
Ostrer, Harry.
Legacy: a genetic history of the Jewish people / Harry Ostrer.
p. cm.
Includes bibliographical references and index.
ISBN 978-0-19-537961-7 (hardcover : alk. paper)
1. Jews.   2. Jews—Origin.   3. Jews—Identity.   I. Title.
GN547.O88 2012
599.98'924—dc23
2011045114

3 5 7 9 8 6 4 2

Printed in the United States of America
on acid-free paper

For Lily, Isabel, and Nathaniel

ACKNOWLEDGMENTS

Clearly, I have benefited from the advice and support of many people, among them the physicians who introduced Tay-Sachs screening and nurtured my Columbia medical school classmate, Madeleine Harbison, and me to set up a Tay-Sachs screening program as our junior public health project in 1975—Stephen Rosenberg, Michael Kaback, Charles Scriver, and Barton Childs. As a medical student, I took the graduate course in human genetics, and I found it so compelling that I took it a second time and then chose a career in human genetics. Among the faculty who taught me were Paul Marks, Richard Rifkind, Arthur Bank, Georgianna Jagiello, and Dorothy Warburton. As a resident and fellow at Johns Hopkins, I benefited from the mentorship of the geneticists

Barton Childs, Haig Kazazian, Victor McKusick, David Valle, Barbara Migeon, and Kirby Smith. I still remember with great fondness the raging lunchtime conversations with Haig and Barbara. At Albert Einstein College of Medicine, I have benefited from the support of my colleagues, Edward Burns, Gil Atzmon, Bernice Morrow, David Reynolds, Michael Prystowski, Jan Vijg, and Allen Spiegel. At NYU School of Medicine, I benefited from the support of my colleagues, Carole Oddoux, Ruth Oratz, Freya Schnabel, Daniel Roses, John Pappas, Felicia Axelrod, and Lauren Carpiniello. My work has benefitted from the financial support of the National Foundation for Jewish Genetic Diseases, the Dysautonomia Foundation, the Jean Batkin Memorial Fund, the Littauer Foundation, Lola Finkelstein, Jack and Susan Rudin, the Lewis and Rachel Rudin Foundation, the Iranian-American Jewish Federation, the Shifrin/Myers Breast Cancer Discovery Fund and the David Himelberg Foundation. In the process of formulating my ideas about the genetics of Jewish peoples, I have profited from discussions with colleagues Neil Risch, Arno Motulsky, Mary-Claire King, Michael Hammer, Karl Skorecki, Doron Behar, Eitan Friedman, Bolek Goldman, Mordechai Shani, Susan Gross, David Goldstein, Neil Bradman, Batsheva Bonne-Tamir, Ariel Darvasi, Ann Pulver, Itsik Pe'er, Carlos Bustamante, David Reich, and Nick Paterson. Paul Marks alerted me to the importance of Chaim Sheba's work and Werner Maas to the importance of Maurice Fishberg's work. Lawrence Shiffman, formerly Chairman of Jewish Studies at NYU and now Vice Provost for Undergraduate Education at Yeshiva University, has often been only a phone call away for setting me straight about Jewish history. Aron Rodrigue and Harvey Goldberg were also very generous in helping me to improve my knowledge of Jewish history.

My daughters, Lily and Isabel, and my late mother, Gloria, aided firsthand in some of my efforts to collect specimens and data from subjects, including members of my family or potential kin. My daughters, my son, Nathaniel, and my wife, Elizabeth Marks, showed remarkable patience, love, and support over the time that it took to complete this manuscript. My agent, Albert Zuckerman, and his wife, Claire, helped me to improve the narrative line. Although I started with a different editor at Oxford University Press, I was fortunate to have Joan Bossert and Chad Zimmerman assigned to me. Their support was critical for promoting the idea of a trade book in Jewish population genetics. Gordon Cook, my illustrator, was a can-do guy with a great eye and a great sense of humor.

CONTENTS

PREFACE

In June 2010, I published a scientific article that demon-strated a biological basis for Jewishness.[1] Using methods that were developed by Itsik Pe'er, a young computer scientist at Columbia University, and others, my collaborators and I showed that the genomes of Jewish people are woven together by a series of DNA threads—not shared among all individuals, because not all Jewish people are the same. This study, termed the *Jewish HapMap Project*, showed that sharing was greater between Iranian Jews or between Ashkenazi (Eastern European) Jews but still discernible between Iranian and Ashkenazi Jews and among all of the Jewish groups examined. Upon probing further, we saw that the history of the Jewish people could be observed in their genomes—founding of populations, population bottlenecks and expansions, conversions, and admixture with non-Jewish peoples. These observations were not casual, because the scientific reviewers of our manuscript, unknown to us through the peer review system of the *American Journal of Human Genetics*, required rigorous analysis through application of stringent statistical methods.

This publication that described the biological basis for Jewishness gained international press coverage and galvanized the public. When we started the study, our clearly stated goal was not to influence public opinion but, rather, to understand the origins and migrations of Jewish peoples. Some have suggested to me that I should seek financial support to promote a political agenda with population genetic analysis, but I have shunned the idea. Some of the commentators sought to rewrite our article for us, suggesting that we didn't get the history quite right or that our scientific methods were flawed. One commentator suggested that the genetic sharing that we observed between Ashkenazi and Sephardic (Southern European) Jews reflected greater than expected interchange and intermarriage between the two communities during medieval times.[2] In fact, the study did not require rewriting. The data were quite compatible with a shared origin in southern Europe for both groups and the well-known fact that the progenitors of Ashkenazi Jews migrated over the Alps into the Rhine Valley during the first millennium of the Common Era. Denying the facts of the study, another commentator suggested that our observations were entirely wrong ("No study...has succeeded in identifying a genetic marker specific to Jews.").[3] In fact, replication of much of our study was published by Skorecki and Behar's group in the scientific journal *Nature* a week later.[4] These investigators went on to characterize other Jewish groups that we had not. The tenor of the debate was turned up when this commentator told journalist Michael Balter that Hitler would have been pleased by our findings. Wow! Despite our considerable effort to use the most rigorous of scientific approaches, the discredited race science theories of the Nazis were cited as proof of our misguided behavior. This imputation of equivalence was morally objectionable, because we were not seeking to develop a hierarchy of human groups nor attempting to eliminate individuals on the basis of their having "undesirable" genes or traits, as the Nazis had. The comments were also uninformed, because human genetics has been moving at a rapid clip in recent years, requiring considerable effort even from human geneticists to keep up. Some commentators later pointed out to me that they were unsure what they had commented about. One even apologized for an insensitive and erroneous remark.

This overheated discussion in the press without dispassionate analysis of scientific observations proved to me that a popular book about Jewish population genetics might tone down the debate into a more thoughtful realm. Notably, it would be useful to review how Jews themselves were once promoters of race science theories that were based on few physical measurements and many preconceived notions. Later, Jewish geneticists championed the emerging field of population genetics but lacked the tools that have become available only in our times. Such books have been written in the past and, yet, none with the benefit of the contemporary methods of population genetics that have defined human populations with a degree of rigor previously unknown. Explaining these methods to develop a common lexicon for population genetics is important, so that commentators can judge the evidence for themselves before weighing in on the debate.

The Jewish HapMap Project was the latest effort in my 25-plus-year career to understand not only the origins and migrations of Jewish people but also their disease susceptibilities. It was my effort as a medical geneticist to bring the benefits of contemporary human genetics to my own people and to understand my Jewishness. For me, the work with various aspects of Jewish genetics provided a new framework for thinking about Jews. At last one could confront head-on the often debated question of whether Jews constituted a race, a people, or a genetic isolate. "Race" was a technical term used by nineteenth-century biologists to describe groups of organisms. Today their use of the term appears quaint. Charles Darwin discussed how interbreeding between races could lead sometimes to sterile offspring.[5] We would now call these *races* "different species." On the other hand, Darwin discussed how interbreeding between races could lead sometimes to fertile offspring with enhanced hybrid vigor. We would term these *races* "varietals" or "breeds." When applied to humans, race has come to mean a group with a characteristic physical appearance, including skin, hair and eye color, skull and facial form, limb length, and stature. The preferred terms in the twenty-first century might be "continental groups" or "ethnic groups," depending on their geographic scopes and histories. At the opposite extreme is the term "genetic isolate," meaning a group that did not reproduce with other groups, either by choice or by geographic isolation. Clearly, this phenomenon occurred for specific Jewish groups during the Diaspora and accounted in part for why certain genetic conditions became prevalent in these groups. Intermarriage has been common at different times during Jewish history. Typically, when Jews intermarried, their children were lost to the faith and to the people. This loss, whether voluntary or involuntary, was reflected by the mourning ritual of *shiva* for the member who married outside the group. Yet, the Jewish contribution to the genetics of the departed offspring was not necessarily lost and could be found in their descendants in southern Africa, in the San Luis Valley of Colorado, and elsewhere in the Old World and New. These "gee whiz" observations have had great appeal to *New York Times* readers and *NOVA* watchers. Some of the aspects of Jewish lore could be validated, most notably evidence for shared ancestry among Jewish men from the Cohanim priestly lineage. Other bits of Jewish lore cannot—the claims for a historical King David can be found only in the archeological record, not in the genetic record despite considerable effort. Thus, the Jews can be said to be a people with a shared genetic legacy, although not all Jews share the same genes, nor is having part of that legacy a requirement for being Jewish. Having a 3000-year genetic legacy can be a source of group identity and pride in the same way that having a shared history, culture, and religion can be sources of pride. Many Jews and non-Jews alike want to know the story of that genetic legacy. Many people try to recreate their own legacies by constructing their genealogies and seeking genetic testing to try to fill in the gaps. Others are content to read or hear the story.

So, in this book, I have tried to tell the story of the genetics of Jewish people. I chose not to be encyclopedic as were the earlier writers, Maurice Fishberg and Richard Goodman, but rather to convey the major storyline. In the process, I may have left out details about specific groups or diseases that merit telling in the future. I have not shied away from controversy, recognizing population genetic claims might fuel territorial stakes, such as the claims of both Jews and Palestinians for homelands in Israel and the West Bank. I have recognized that genetic insights might fire up new debates about the purported superiority of one group over another. I have also considered that genetic determinants may give one group a larger burden of disease predisposition, such as cancer and depression. Originally I had thought to write the narratives of patients and genealogists, but I rapidly discarded this approach in favor of writing the narratives of the scientists and physicians who made the discoveries, because I learned from reading Stephen Jay Gould and Armand Marie Leroi that their stories could be compelling.[6–7] I have tried not only to make the narratives interesting but also to make the genetics accessible to the general reader, without diluting any of the content.

ONE

LOOKING JEWISH

At the turn of the twentieth century, New York City was the largest Jewish city in the world. Among the almost 1 million Jews were many professional and business people who had attained prominence in medicine, law, finance, media, entertainment, and the garment industry. Some readily assimilated into the melting pot of cosmopolitan New York, whereas others clung boldly to their Jewish identity. Who were the Jews anyway? Were they a race of people whose lineage had been maintained since Biblical times? Could they be identified by their looks? Why did certain diseases seem to cluster among them? Maurice Fishberg, a young Russian Jewish immigrant physician, grappled with the issues of Jewish origins, identity, and traits in a series of papers that culminated in a book,

The Jews: A Study of Race and Environment.[8–9] Today, Fishberg's work retains an uncanny freshness on the issues of identity that continue to confront contemporary Jews and non-Jews alike.

Fishberg was a typical socially mobile Jewish immigrant, much like the people that he catalogued (Figure I.I).[10–12] Born Mordecai Yehuda Fishberg in 1872, in the town of Kanenetz-Podolsk, Russia, he came to the United States at the age of 17 years, during the great wave of Eastern European

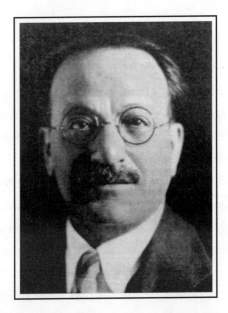

Figure I.I. Maurice Fishberg, American physical anthropologist and author of *The Jews: a Study of Race and Environment*. Fishberg was criticized by his contemporaries for not considering the Jews to be a race.

Jewish immigration. Like many immigrants, he aspired to study at an American university, but upon his arrival in New York he found that his Russian public school diploma was insufficient to meet entrance requirements. As he told an interviewer for the Yiddish newspaper, *Der Tog*, in 1925, "If you are hungry, you can do anything."[10] He worked at a variety of jobs, including coal mining for 6 months in Pennsylvania. Although backbreaking work, this coal mining job left him with time in the evenings to study English, mathematics, and other subjects that were required for admission to a university. After completing this period of self-study (and coal mining), Fishberg was accepted to the New York University School of Medicine and returned to New York.

In 1897, Fishberg obtained a medical degree and opened a practice on the Lower East Side of Manhattan. Practicing medicine in a poor community was a difficult way to earn a living, so the newly graduated Dr. Fishberg supplemented his income with moonlighting jobs at the Tombs Prison, the New York City Health Department, and the New York Life Insurance Company. In 1901, these odd jobs led to a position as the chief medical examiner for the United Hebrew Charities, which he held for 14 years, assessing the well-being of newly arrived immigrants. This job provided Fishberg with financial security and a platform for his roles as a medical advocate and physical anthropologist—his interest was both practical and academic. As a medical advocate, he confronted immigration restriction supporters who claimed that the Jews brought communicable diseases, especially tuberculosis (TB), into the United States. He noted:

> Many writers on the racial effects of the recent immigration have alleged that 'inferior' racial elements are likely to dete- riorate physically the people of the United States... None of these writers to my knowledge made an effort to study the problem directly from the strictly scientific standpoint, so that their statements on the subject can be considered merely opinions not necessarily based on facts.[13]

Fishberg demonstrated the fallacy of the argument that Jews brought TB into the United States in a 1901 paper that he published in *American Medicine*.[14] As urban dwellers with rela- tively small chest cavities, crowded living conditions, and indoor occupations, such as tailoring, they might have been expected to have a higher frequency of TB than the population at large. When Fishberg examined the U.S. census and New York Board of Health data on consumption (TB) as a cause of death, he observed that the rate was far lower among Jews than among other immigrant groups and native-born Americans (Figure 1.2). He also observed that the lower death rate from consumption was not peculiar to Jews living in the United States but also occurred among Jews living in London, Tunis, and Australia. Fishberg attributed the Jews' lower susceptibility to TB to lifestyle factors, such as eating kosher meat from care- fully inspected animals and to the infrequency of risk factors such as syphilis and alcoholism.

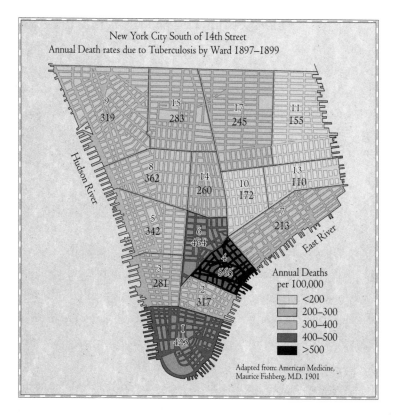

Figure I.2. Fishberg's map of annual tuberculosis death rates by ward in
New York City south of 14th Street 1897–1899. Note that the rates
were lowest in the wards that had the highest proportion of
Jews—the 10th, 11th, and 13th. (See color figure.)

Fishberg went on to explore the prevalence of other diseases
in the Jewish population to bolster his arguments that Jewish
immigration would not lead to the degeneration of the U.S.
population. In the process, he pulled together vital statistics and

health data for various groups in the United States, Europe, and North Africa.[15] His conclusion about *enhanced* life-expectancy among Jews was striking. "All over Europe, whenever tested, the Jews have been found, in spite of their frail physical aspect, to live longer than the Christians." In Budapest, the life expectancy was 37 years for Jews and 26 years for Christians. In London, the life expectancy was 49 years for Jews and 37 years for Christians. Both marriage and birth rates were lower among Jews than among neighboring Christian populations, yet this longevity led to a higher rate of population growth caused by lower death rates among the Jews. The death rates were lower for several epidemic diseases, including smallpox and cholera. This lower death rate from cholera occurred not only in Europe (Budapest) but also in North Africa (Algiers). Organic diseases of the brain and spinal cord, resulting from alcoholism and syphilis, were also less common among Jews.

Jews were not immune to all diseases. Diabetes was very common, accounting for 25% of the deaths from this disease in New York City (at a time when the Jewish population was only 20% of the city's total). In fact, diabetes was called a *Judenkrankheit*, a Jewish disease, by some German physicians. Fishberg disagreed with this analysis and noted, "On the whole there is no justification for considering diabetes a racial disease of the Jews. It has not been observed to be more frequent among the Jews in every country than among their non-Jewish neighbours."[8] He observed that mental illness and mental retardation were more common than diabetes among Jews. In his parlance, "the Jews

Table I.I. Average annual number of insane during 1890–1902 per 100,000 population and the forms of insanity with which they were affected.

Form	Christians	Jews
Congenital idiocy	0.7	0.98
Congenital imbecility	2.05	3.53
Melancholia	2.97	3.89
Mania	1.61	3.87
Amentia	7.62	13.44
Paranoia	5.41	5.96
Psychosis periodica	1.99	4.86
Dementia	6.79	10.79
Progressive paralysis	7.77	11.07
Epileptic insanity	3.1	2.22
Hysterical insanity	1.35	2.04
Insanity, with neurasthenia	0.71	1.78
Psychosis cum cerebropathiacircumscripta	0.45	0.62
Psychosis cum pellagra	0.5	0.16
Alcoholism	5.44	0.68
Alcoholism, with drug addiction	0.14	0.28
Other forms	0.65	1.42

Adapted with permission from M. Fishberg, *The Jews: A Study of Race and Environment.* New York: Charles Scribner's Sons, 1911, p. 346.

supply proportionately two to five more mental defectives than the Christians" (Table I.I).[15] The higher frequencies of insanity and idiocy among Jews had a wide geographic distribution and were reported in Italy, Germany, and Russia. Similarly, functional neuroses, which bore the now quaint names of "hysteria" and "neurasthenia," were markedly more common among Jews.

He reported that amaurotic family idiocy (a progressive neurodegenerative condition now known as "Tay-Sachs disease") occurred almost exclusively among Jews.

Fishberg delved into various reasons why certain conditions might be more prevalent among Jews. He claimed:

> The causes of the peculiarities of the comparative pathology of the Jews have at different times received different interpretations. Some have attributed the fact that the Jews have a longer duration of life, a lower mortality, etc, and also their greater liability to be affected with nervous diseases than non-Jews, to indolence of the Jew, to his lack of exercise, to the rich, highly seasoned food that the Jews are supposed to eat…That the Jews are obliged to keep two Sundays a week…about twice as many leisure days as Christians is another argument. But all these reasons do not hold good at present, particularly with our American Jews, as almost everybody who comes in contact with modern Jews will testify.[8]

He also rejected consanguinity (the marriage of Jews to close relatives, including aunts, uncles, and cousins) as an explanation. But Fishberg's view that consanguineous marriages among healthy individuals are not sometimes deleterious to posterity would not withstand the test of time. Fishberg realized that Jews might present a unique opportunity to study the roles of nature and nurture in human development and disease. As he noted:

> The study of the somatic characteristics of the Jews has received the attention of many anthropologists in Europe.

It was suggested that because they have kept themselves socially isolated for nearly two thousand years, and have refrained from intermarriage with other races, the Jews offer a promising field for the solution of many obscure problems in the study of man. Considering that they have been scattered over almost every part of the habitable globe; by involuntary and most forced migrations from city to city, country to country and from continent to continent, have been subjected to frequent changes in their physical environment, it was expected that a thorough study of their racial characteristics may contribute to our meager knowledge of the influence of environment upon race. If the Jews have really maintained themselves for the last four thousand years in absolute purity, the effects of climate, attitude, nourishment, economic and social conditions, should be ascertainable by a study of their physical organization. If on the other hand, they have intermarried with races among whom they have dwelt, of if more extensive conversion to Judaism have taken place, and the modern Jews are thus a mixture of various racial elements, blended together in a more or less homogeneous group of people, they should offer excellent material for the study of the effects of racial intermixture on the physical organization of man.[16]

With this idea, Fishberg launched his next career as a physical anthropologist.

Fishberg was not the first to tackle this question, as the field of race science was in full flourish at this time. Both theories of Jewish origins—ethnic purity and racial composite—were popular. He framed the issue in this way,

> From the comparative large number of measurements taken on living subjects, authorities have drawn different conclusions. Some...have maintained that the Jews are a pure race, the descendants of the primitive Semites, and almost entirely unmixed with foreign blood, while others have stated that the results of the study of the physical characteristics of the Jews are against this view.[17]

The basis for drawing these conclusions was anthropometry—the measurement and comparison of physical traits, such as head form and pigmentation, of individuals thought to comprise distinctive groups (Figure 1.3). Head form was thought to be a racial characteristic minimally influenced by environment, nutrition, or social selection. The rules for calculating head form as a "cephalic index" were fairly precise. The cephalic index was calculated by first measuring the length, the diameter of the head from the forehead to the most distant point of the occiput, then the width at the widest diameter behind the temples. The width multiplied by 100 divided by the length equals the cephalic index. To minimize error, the measurements were repeated, and the mean of two measurements was recorded. Fishberg based his analyses on the measurements that he made on more than 4,000 Jews of European origin in New York City and on the published results of Jews residing in European countries (Figure 1.4). He observed that

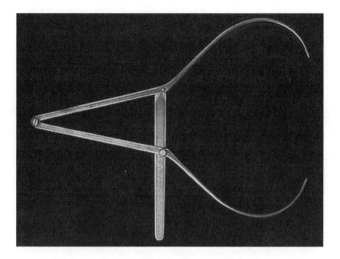

Figure I.3. Calipers similar to those used by Maurice Fishberg and
other physical anthropologists for measuring head proportions to
determine cephalic indices. (See color figure.)

most European Jews had a cephalic index of between 81 and
83, making them round-headed, or "brachycephalic." When he
plotted his results for Jewish men graphically, he observed a
curve with a single peak and fairly narrow width, suggesting
a homogeneous distribution. Fishberg was impressed by these
results, noting, "Such homogeneity of the cranial type has
not been observed in any other civilized race."[17] Yet, for reasons that he could not explain, the cephalic index distribution
of Jewish women generated a curve that almost completely
overlapped that of men but had two peaks, suggesting two
possible groups.

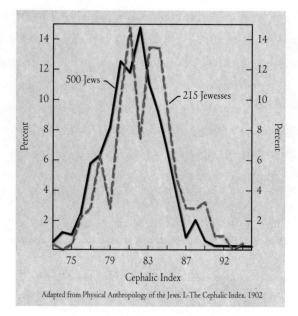

Adapted from Physical Anthropology of the Jews. I.-The Cephalic Index, 1902

Figure I.4. Fishberg's graphs for the cephalic indices of Jewish men and women. A cephalic index of 81–83 is indicative of brachycephaly or round-headedness. Note that the Jewish men had a curve with a single peak and fairly narrow width, suggesting a homogeneous distribution. The cephalic index distribution for Jewish women almost completely overlapped that of men but had two peaks, suggesting two possible groups. (See color figure.)

The second trait that Fishberg studied was pigmentation. He deemed the color of skin, hair, and eyes to be a very important racial trait but took into consideration the influences of climate, altitude, nutrition, and social class.[18] Fishberg observed that dark pigmentation is common among Jews. In his investigation of 2,272 Jews in New York City, including 1,188 men and 1,084 women, he found that 80% of the men and women had dark hair. Yet, in another gender-based paradox, Fishberg observed that 77% of the men had light skin and 65% of the women had dark skin. Physical anthropologists in European countries found different proportions of dark-haired and dark-skinned men and women. Fishberg took this as evidence of racial admixture, while still raising the question of whether the progenitor stock in Palestine included individuals with light hair and skin or whether Jews were derived by admixture or conversion of other peoples during the long history of Diaspora. Fishberg noted:

> One of the most important problems in the anthropology of the Jews had been the origin of the Jews with fair hair and eyes, and it has been discussed by everyone who wrote on the subject. Generally speaking, two theories have been advanced. One…is to the effect that the blond Jews have their origin in intermixture with Northern European races. Others claim, however, that blondness is no proof of intermixture with Teutonic races of Europe. As has been mentioned, there were blonde Jews in Biblical times, and the modern blonde Jews are considered as descendents of the blondes at the time of the Bible.[8]

This issue is still the subject of considerable debate almost 100 years later.

After his extensive fieldwork and analysis, Fishberg came to the conclusion that the Jews were not a pure race but a racial composite, having mixed with surrounding populations during their long history. There were no enduring racial differences between Jews and the non-Jews among whom they lived. "Jews bear a striking resemblance to the ethnic types encountered in the indigenous races and peoples among whom they happen to live. Moreover, only a small proportion of the European Jews display the traits which are said to be characteristic of the other Semitic races living to-day in Asia and Africa."[19] Having derived these conclusions, Fishberg decided to examine the Jews of Algeria and Tunis to determine whether they resembled the Jews of Europe or the local populations. The North African Jews appeared taller, darker, and longer-headed than their European brethren. Nonetheless, fair Jews with round heads were observed in both populations, albeit at a higher frequency among the European Jews. Fishberg dispelled the stereotype of hooked noses— finding them to be, in fact, rare among European Jews and rarer still among North African Jews. So by 1906, Fishberg decided that there was no such thing as a Jewish race. Jews varied physically by country of origin and even by provinces within one country. Jews were tall and short, blond and brunette, brachycephalic and dolichocephalic, in the same way that Catholics and Protestants in European countries showed considerable variation.[9]

Fishberg, nonetheless, perceived the presence of a Jewish physiognomy, or look, and filled his book with photographs of Jews from all over the world, who, to his eye, resembled one another. As he said, "One can pick out a Jew from among a thousand non-Jews without difficulty."[8] The idea of looking Jewish was championed by Fishberg's contemporary, Joseph Jacobs, the leading Jewish physical anthropologist in England at the time and a proponent of the view that Jews constituted a single race. In 1901, Jacobs came to America to become the Revising Editor of the *Jewish Encyclopedia*, the compendium of Jewish history, literature, and theology of the time. In his article on anthropology, Jacobs noted, "The remarkable unity of resemblance among Jews, even in different climes, seems to imply a common descent. Photographs of Jews taken in Bokhara resemble almost to identity those of Jews in Berlin or New York."[20] Jacobs thought that countenance, or expression, was conserved among Jews even when head-form was not. Jacobs suggested that there might be a genetic basis for looking Jewish and, evoking the newly discovered science of genetics, he suggested that it might even be a dominant trait! "Wherever such a type had been socially or racially selected, the law of inheritance discovered by G. Mendel would imply that any hybrids tend to revert to it, and a certain amount of evidence has been given for the prepotency of the Jewish side in mixed marriages." The idea of looking Jewish lingered over the course of the twentieth century. Joseph Epstein, a columnist writing for the *Weekly Standard*, 90 years after Jacob's theory, noted, "And yet Jews remain, at least to most other Jews, identifiably, unmistakably Jewish."[21] The idea of looking Jewish resonated outside the Jewish community. In the 1980s, the Doyle Dane Bernbach advertising agency conducted a successful and humorous campaign showing the portrait of an Indian chief with the caption, "You don't have to be Jewish to love Levy's rye bread," implying that everyone in America knows how Jews should look.

Jacobs acknowledged that the issue of homogeneity of Jewish ancestry was unresolved. He also acknowledged that the stakes were large for Zionism—the proposed creation of a Jewish homeland in Palestine, which was another important issue of the time. If the Jews were not a race but a people, then they had no claim to a geographic ancestral homeland.[22]

Fishberg's views encountered some heated opposition in New York because he refuted the popular view that Jews constituted a distinct race. The anonymous book reviewer in *The New York Times* wrote, "Dr. Fishberg seems most anxious to make his own people as commonplace as possible and to rob them of all claim to the title of a peculiar people." Yet, citing Fishberg's own evidence, the reviewer questioned whether his conclusion was warranted: "If the shape of the skull depends on habitat rather than race, Dr. Fishberg's elaborate measurements go by the board and do not prove his contention of intermixture of the Jewish race, for which there is little evidence."[23] In a letter to the editor of the *Times*, Annette Kohn questioned the sufficiency of Fishberg's arguments. "Certain it is that it needs a wider discussion and the production of more evidence in proof than the Doctor has given to have his facts accepted. Heretofore the world has accepted a theory in direct opposition to his conclusions."[24]

The concept of race, identifiable by the traits of skin, hair and eye color, skull and facial form, limb length, and height, seemed very clear to people living a century ago.[8] What seemed clear a century ago has become murky and contentious today.

In a recent special supplement of the journal *Nature Genetics*, dedicated to genetics and race, Jorde and Wooding wrote:

Few concepts have as tarnished and contentious a history as "race." Among both the scientific and lay communities, the notion that humans can be grouped into different races has been enshrined by some and dismissed by others. Even the definition of race varies considerably, depending on context and criteria...Not surprisingly, biomedical scientists are divided in their opinions about race. Some characterize it as "biologically meaningless" or "not based on scientific evidence," whereas others advocate the use of race in making decisions about medical treatment or the design of research studies.[25]

Writing in the same issue, Tishkoff and Kidd built on these views: "One of the problems with using 'race' as an identifier is the lack of a clear definition of race."[26] Much like Fishberg and Jacobs, they noted that race was based on body size and shape, skin color, language, culture, religion, ethnicity, and geographic origin. Body size and shape and skin color were not good indicators because they could be influenced by adaptation to environmental conditions. People who were exposed to similar environmental conditions may have converged to look alike—people with dark skin are found in New Guinea, Southern India, and Africa, despite these groups having had little or no contact with each other over thousands of years. Culture, language, religion, and ethnicity may be acquired and are not necessarily indicators of shared ancestry—people who

LEGACY

are called Latino in the United States include individuals of European, Native American, and African ancestry in all possible combinations. Geographic origins of people may not be synonymous with race because of recent, historical, and prehistorical migrations.

Yet a consensus view has emerged that is shared by these contemporary geneticists and others. Risch and his co-authors explained this consensus view in an influential article in the journal *Genome Biology.*

> Probably the best way to examine the issue of genetic subgrouping is through the lens of human evolution. If the human population mated at random, there would be no issue of genetic subgrouping because the chance of any individual carrying a specific gene variant would be evenly distributed around the world. For a variety of reasons, however, including geography, sociology and culture, humans have not and do not currently mate randomly, either on a global level or within countries such as the U.S.[27]

They went on to note that human populations originated in Africa and that groups outside Africa were derived from migration events out of Africa that occurred within the last 100,000 years. Because of their long-term residence in Africa, perhaps antedating the migration events by 150,000 years, the greatest genetic variation occurs within Africans. Variation outside Africa represents a subset of African diversity, or variants that arose after the migration. Between individuals, genetic differentiation depends on the degree and duration of separation of their ancestors. Genetic differentiation is enhanced by geographic isolation and by inbreeding (endogamy) over extended periods of time and is reduced by mating between populations. As a result, many human population genetic studies have shown that the greatest genetic differentiation occurs on a continental basis. These studies have recapitulated the classical definition of races based on continental ancestry—African, Caucasian (Europe and Middle East), Asian, Pacific Islander (Australian, New Guinean, and Melanesian), and Native American. Tishkoff and Kidd simplified this view even further:

> Some argue that there is no such thing as 'race' or that it is biologically meaningless. Yet the lay person will ridicule that position as nonsense, because people from different parts of the world look different, whereas people from the same part of the world tend to look similar.[26]

So "looking Jewish" should reflect the common geographic origin of contemporary Jewish people with evidence of a shared genetic legacy among themselves.

Viewed in the context of Jewish history, the genetic makeup of contemporary Jewish populations has been influenced by the geographic origins of a relatively small number of founders. The makeup of these populations has been further influenced by migration (giving rise to a new group of founders), admixture with neighboring populations, and variation in the rate of population growth at different times of Jewish history. The original

founders are thought to have been Semitic nomads whose stories are described in the Bible.[28] The patriarchs, Abraham, Isaac
and Jacob; the matriarchs, Sarah, Rebecca, Leah, and Rachel;
and their entourage gave rise to 12 tribes and, in turn, two
kingdoms. The accuracy of Biblical sources has been called into
question by some contemporary historians,[29] but the discovery in 1991 of an old inscribed stone in the town of Tel Dan,
Israel, provided archeological evidence for a Jewish kingdom
that was ruled by the Biblical King David and his descendants.
This stone dated from 825 B.C.E. and had 13 lines of Aramaic
script that celebrated the defeat of Josephat of Judah," King of
the House of David," by King Hadad II of Aram-Damascus.
This stone, known as "the House of David Inscription," is dis-
played at the Israel Museum in Jerusalem.[30]

Following the destruction of the Jewish kingdoms more
than 2,000 years ago, the Jews became a migratory people who
established communities throughout the world.[31] Some of these
communities retained their continuity over long periods of
time. Within those communities, Jews were linked by religion,
customs, marriage, and language (often a Jewish dialect of a
local language). The designation "Jewish" was limited by religious law to those whose mothers were Jewish. Entry into the
community was possible through religious conversion, but this
was not common. Jewish identity was maintained within these
communities up to present day.

Most contemporary Jewish populations are affiliated with
one of four groups that are determined by place of immigration

and long-term residence. Middle Eastern (or Mizrahi) Jews lived in contemporary Israel and Palestine, as well as in Iran, Iraq, Central Asia, and the Arabian Peninsula. The progenitors of the Iraqi, Iranian, and Central Asian populations were forcibly carried into captivity in Babylon (in present-day Iraq) following the destruction of the first Jewish Temple in 586 B.C.E. (This was the second of the major exiles. The first occurred in 722 B.C.E., when 27,290 members of the Kingdom of Israel were deported by the Assyrian king. This later gave rise to myths about the contribution of the "Ten Lost Tribes" that comprised this kingdom to the formation of Ethiopian Jews, Indian Jews, English, Japanese, Native Americans, and many other groups.) Sephardic Jews (from the Hebrew word for "Spanish") resided in Spain and Portugal under both Moslem and Christian rule. At the time of the Spanish Inquisition in the late fifteenth century, Jews who did not convert to Christianity were expelled from Spain and later from Portugal. These Jews migrated to North Africa, Italy, the Balkans, Turkey, Lebanon, Syria, and the Americas.[32] The Sephardic Jews of Turkey and the Balkans spoke Ladino, a Jewish dialect of Spanish, a tradition that was not necessarily maintained by other Sephardic Jews. The Ashkenazi Jews (from the Hebrew word for "German") moved north of the Alps, probably from Italy, during the first millennium of the Common Era.[33] During the ninth century, the ancestors of Ashkenazi Jews settled in the cities of the Rhineland, where they adopted German as their language. Over time, this developed into a Judeo-German dialect that was relexified with Hebrew and Slavic words and became known as "Yiddish." In the twelfth and thirteenth centuries, Ashkenazi Jews were expelled from the countries of Western Europe and were granted charters to settle in Poland and Lithuania. As a result, the center of Ashkenazi Jewry shifted to the East, where it remained for the following five centuries. The North African Jews resided along the coast of North Africa for more than two millennia.[34] The Jewish populations of Libya, Tunisia, Algeria, and Morocco are descended from Israelite traders who colonized the coast along with Phoenician traders, exiles who left Palestine following the destruction of the Temples, and local converts, often from Berber tribes. The Jewish populations thrived in Roman times, having left a rich archeological trove of synagogues and mosaics. The Jewish chronicler Josephus reported the presence of 500,000 Jews in Cyrenaica alone in the first century C.E., although these communities did not thrive for much of their history under Arab and Ottoman rule.

Admixture with surrounding populations had a role in shaping the face of world Jewry. Fishberg noted:

> The greatest mixtures of which there are any historical records have been taken during the Greco-Roman period of the Jews. Notwithstanding the fact that Judaism is such an exclusive religion, and thought always to discourage proselytism, still during that period it made many converts. Everything points to an intense activity in spreading Judaism among the pagans.[8]

In 141 B.C.E., Jonathan, the brother of Judah Maccabee, established a new Jewish kingdom in Judea. This story of the overthrow of the Greek Selucid kings, the political successors to Alexander the Great, is retold every year during the holiday of Chanukah and is recorded in the Biblical books of the Maccabees. The Hasmonean dynasty (the name of the dynasty was taken from an ancestor of the Maccabees) expanded the kingdom of Judea, so that what had once been a small isolated province in the empires of Cyrus the Great and Alexander the Great became a significant political entity that included much of modern Israel, southern Lebanon, and western Jordan. Simon's son, John Hyrcanus, conquered the peoples of Samaria and Galilee to the north and the Idumea to the south. In the process, he converted the whole population to Judaism and established the Judaization of the whole of Palestine as a permanent element of Hasmonean policy.[28] Although the numbers of people converted is not known, Judea remained a country with a Jewish majority for centuries after the fall of the Hasmonean dynasty in Roman times.[31]

Writing in 1901 about the Diaspora in the *Jewish Encyclopedia*, Gottheil and Reinach noted:

The fervor of proselytism was indeed one of the most distinctive traits of Judaism during the Greco-Roman epoch—a trait which it never possessed in the same degree either before or since. This zeal to make converts, which at first sight seems to be incompatible with the pride of the "chosen people" and with the contempt which the orthodox Jew professed for the foreigner.[35]

The writers went on to note that various methods were used to increase the Jewish population, including both John Hyrcanus's and Aristobulus's forced conversions with circumcision imposed on the Idumeans and on a subgroup of the Itureans (Galileans), respectively. Slaves were forcibly converted. Yet, moral propaganda in speeches, examples, and books was also successful. Despite the use of circumcision and the absence of pagan ritual and sensuous rites, Judaism had a wide appeal. Among the attractive features were the practical and legal character of Jewish doctrine that provided a rule for every occasion, a pure and simple theology, mysterious and quaint customs, an enforced day of Sabbath rest, and certain political privileges. People from both upper and lower classes were successfully proselytized, especially in Egypt, Cyprus, and Syria. As a result, the Jewish population of the Roman Empire grew to comprise 10% of the total, with Egypt, Syria, and Palestine each having a Jewish population of 1 million people (Figure 1.5).

Admixture with other populations occurred at later times during Jewish history. According to Fishberg, "The most important infusion of non-Jewish racial elements into the veins of Eastern European Jews took place in the eighth century when the Chozars adopted Judaism."[8] The Chozars (or Khazars) were a people of Central Asian Turkic origin who ruled a Jewish state between the Caucasus Mountains

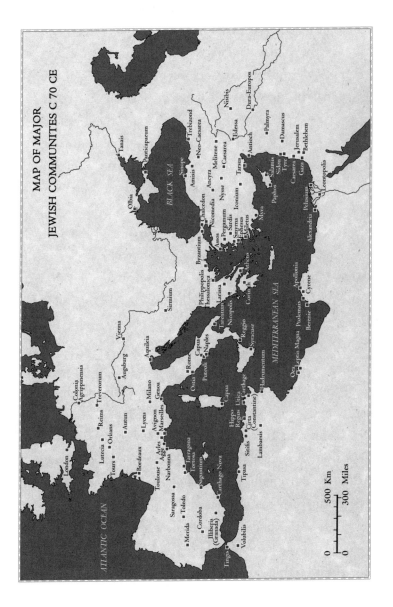

Figure I.5. Map of major Jewish communities circa 70 C.E. These communities spanned the Mediterranean Basin and stretched into Europe and Asia Minor. (See color figure.)

and the Volga River. They spoke a language in a family of languages that includes Turkish, Kazakh, Uzbek, Uigur, and Kirghiz, not the Slavic languages. Their kingdom, established in most of southern Russia long before the rise of the Russian monarchy, acted as a barrier against the northern advance of the Arabs, then at the height of their expansion. This kingdom flourished for two or three centuries, subjugating other tribes in its region and forcing some of its Slavic neighbors to pay tolls for the use of the commercial routes that it controlled. In the middle of the eighth century, the Khazar king and aristocracy embraced Judaism. Ordinary Khazars retained their traditional beliefs and eventually were converted to Islam or Christianity. Around 965 c.e., the Russians overcame the Khazars, destroying their capital and other cities.[33]

The fate of the Khazarian Jews, following the destruction of their kingdom, has been the subject of much speculation. The last of the Khazar kings, George Tzula, was taken prisoner. Some of the Khazars fled to the Crimea, Hungary, and even Spain, but the great mass of the people remained in their native country. In 1976, the Hungarian-English novelist Arthur Koestler published a book, *The Thirteenth Tribe*, in which he advanced the controversial thesis that the masses of Ashkenazi Jews were not descended from the Israelites of antiquity via Italy and the Rhineland but rather from Khazars who moved westward into current Russia, Ukraine, and Poland. Of Ashkenazi Jewish origin himself, Koestler framed the issue this way: "How important, in quantitative terms is the 'presence' of the sons of Japeth (Caucasians) in the tents of tents of Shem (Semites)?"[36] Part of his intent in writing the book was to defuse anti-Semitism by undermining the identification of European Jews with Bibical Jews. Anti-Semitic epithets such as "Christ killer" would be inapplicable to Ashkenazi Jews if they did not have a Semitic origin. Ironically, Koestler's thesis gained currency with anti-Semitic groups who believed that identifying most Jews as non-Semitic would seriously undermine their historical claims to the land of Israel.

Admixture has also been a feature of recent Jewish history. Fishberg observed, "A study of available statistics shows that there are more mixed marriages contracted between Jews and Christians than is generally supposed."[8] In Scandinavia, Hamburg, and Berlin, mixed marriages were almost as common as pure marriages. In the German Empire from 1901 to 1907, mixed marriages constituted 19% of all Jewish marriages. In cities such as Amsterdam, known to have sizable Orthodox populations, mixed marriage was common. In Amsterdam, mixed marriages constituted 9% of Jewish marriages during 1899 to 1901 and 15% of Jewish marriages between 1902 and 1903. Fishberg went on to note that admixture can result in assimilation. By way of example, he noted that the Spanish and Portuguese Jews in England had practically disappeared, having been absorbed through intermarriage with Christians. Intermarriage continues to have a significant impact on Jewish demography. In many Western countries, the rate of intermarriage between Jews and non-Jews is as high as 50%.[37] In Israel, many Jews marry other Jews who are not members of their own historical communities.

Fishberg and his contemporaries appreciated that, in fact, not all Jews resemble one another. In his survey of world Jewry, Fishberg observed that the Black Jews of India, Chinese Jews, and Ethiopian Jews did not look typically Jewish.[8] The *Black* Jews of India lived in Cochin on the Malabar Coast and in Bombay. In both places, they were said to have been the descendants of slaves who were owned by *White* Jews and underwent conversion. Fishberg found Chinese Jews to be "most curious," because they "do not look like Jews at all, but can easily pass as Chinamen." He went on to cite a source who opined that Chinese Jews were the descendents of immigrants from Persia and Central Asia who, over time, "were absorbed by indigenous populations and left no trace behind." Likewise, he noted that in Abyssinia (Ethiopia), there was a large group of Jews, called Falashas, "who are of pure African type." Fishberg observed, "Many of them are black, and have thick lips, which are upturned, and are practically Negroes. They speak the same language, live in similar houses, and have most of the habits of life and customs of the non-Jewish Abyssinians, from whom they differ only in religion." In their origins story, they claimed descent from the retinue of Menelik, the son of King Solomon and the Queen of Sheba.

Besides having founders who migrated and admixed at different rates with local groups, Jewish populations have grown and contracted at different rates within their places of residence, an issue that Fishberg confronted in the opening of *The Jews.*[8] The Bible placed the number of adult males at Mount Sinai at 611,730, implying a total population of more than 3 million. The census of King David counted 1.3 million males older than age 20 years. This figure implied a total population of 5 million, a number that was not achieved again until the nineteenth century and would have meant that the Jewish population density was similar to that of contemporary Israel or Belgium. Following the Babylonian exile in 586 B.C.E., the total number of Jews may not have exceeded 100,000, whereas during Greco-Roman times, the population may have numbered as many as 6 million (Figure 1.6). The world Jewish population

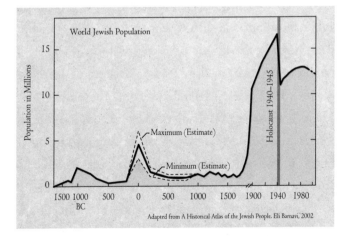

Figure 1.6. Changes in Jewish population size over time. The Jewish population numbered 6 million in Classical Antiquity, a number that was not matched again until the 1800s. (See color figure.)

reached a second nadir during the Middle Ages. Citing the statistics of Benjamin of Tudela, a noted Jewish traveler of the twelfth century, Joseph Jacobs noted that there were "probably no more than 750,000 Jews at the time."[38]

By the beginning of the twentieth century, there were 12 million Jews in the world, of whom 9 million lived in Europe (Figure 1.7).[8] The greatest concentration of Jews (7 million) lived in just three countries—Russia, Austria-Hungary, and Germany—Poland having been divided and annexed by those three countries in the late eighteenth century. According to the 1897 census, 5.1 million Jews lived in Russia, of whom 3.6 million lived in the Pale of Settlement, a region designated for Jewish settlement that was comprised of 15 provinces in the west of European Russia. Another 1.3 million Jews lived in the region of Poland that Russia annexed during the late eighteenth century. According to the 1900 census, 1.2 million Jews lived in Austria-Hungary, two-thirds of whom resided in Galicia—the part of Poland partitioned by Austria. According to the 1905 census, 607,000 Jews lived in Germany, of whom 409,000 resided in Prussia as a result of the annexation of Polish territory. These turn-of-the-century censuses demonstrated that the majority of Jews who resided in Europe were descendants of the fourteenth century founders of Polish Jewry. Through the wave of late nineteenth and early twentieth century immigration, these Ashkenazi Jews came to comprise the majority Jewish population in the United States, Canada, South America, South Africa, Australia, and the United Kingdom. For the most part,

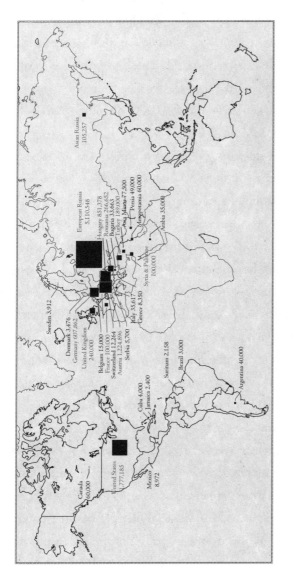

Figure 1.7. Map of major Jewish communities circa 1900 C.E. The sizes of the squares correspond to the sizes of the Jewish populations. Virtually all Diaspora communities were still inhabited by Jews. Almost 2 million Jews lived in the United States by that time. (See color figure.)

Asian Russia 105,257

European Russia 5,110,548

Hungary 851,378
Romania 266,652
Bulgaria 33,663
Turkey 189,000
Asia Minor 77,500
Persia 49,000
Mesopotamia 60,000

Arabia 35,000

Syria & Palestine 100,000

Sweden 3,912
Denmark 3,476
Germany 607,862
United Kingdom 240,000
Belgium 15,000
France 100,000
Switzerland 12,264
Austria 1,224,896
Serbia 5,700
Italy 35,617
Greece 8,350

Surinam 2,158
Brazil 3,000

Cuba 4,000
Jamaica 2,400

Argentina 40,000

Canada 60,000

United States 1,777,185

Mexico 8,972

these were the Jews about whom Fishberg, Jacobs, and others studied and wrote. By 1905, the 762,000 Jews living in New York City comprised 20% of the city's population, making it the largest Jewish city in the world. Jewish populations in other locales were smaller. In the early twentieth century, the total population of Asian Jewry was 500,000, including 250,000 in Palestine and Asia Minor.[8]

In Fishberg's snapshot of Jewish life in 1911, Jews lived in many different communities around the world, most of which have vanished through migration or the Holocaust. The diversity of Diaspora Jewish cultural life, so well catalogued by Fishberg, has been lost with the communities. Today, most Jews live in the United States and Israel, but in 1911 most Jews lived in Eastern and Southern Europe, North Africa, and the Middle East and Central Asia. In Russia, the Jews lived under an oppressive Czarist regime without civil rights. Yet, their oppression was a cohesive force for maintaining their adherence to the community and the faith. As a group, Russian Jews married early and had large families. The high growth rate led to a tripling of this population during the nineteenth century.

By contrast, their Westernized co-religionists—often their relatives—demonstrated behavior that is typical of middle-class people: later marriage, smaller families, and a far greater tendency to intermarry and assimilate. The rates of intermarriage for the Jews of Western and Central Europe exceeded 50%, just as they do for Westernized Jews today. In the West and in Russia, they were most commonly employed in the garment trade. Young Western Jews attended universities in record numbers, many commonly studying law and medicine. Put into context, those garment workers were our great-grandparents, and the middle-class professionals were our grandparents.

In 1911, the forces of social cohesion were religion, race science, and Zionism. Often, race science and Zionism went hand-in-hand, and the identification of a Jewish race provided justification for an ancestral homeland. This issue was addressed head-on in the Paris Peace Conference of 1919, and the consensus on a Jewish race led to the mandate for the creation of a Jewish state in Palestine.

So the Jewish world of 1911 is the predecessor of the Jewish world of the twenty-first century. Many of the Diaspora communities are gone and, as Fishberg predicted, the center of Jewish life has moved to the United States and to Israel. The issues that preoccupied the Jewish intellectual leaders of 1911 are the same ones that preoccupy the leaders of today. Who are the Jews, a religious group or a genetic isolate? Did they originate from Middle Eastern matriarchs and patriarchs? Fishberg lacked the tools for answering these questions. The genetic methods that would eventually provide answers were starting to develop in Fishberg's New York in the Columbia University laboratory of Thomas Hunt Morgan. The precision of these genetic tools continued to improve over the course of the twentieth century, and as they did, Fishberg's intellectual heirs sought to apply them to the issues of Jewish origins and identity.

TWO

FOUNDERS

Chaim Sheba was a colorful, pioneering Israeli geneticist, who was also a surgeon general of the Israeli Army and director general of the Israeli Ministry of Health (Figure 2.1). In June 1961, while serving as the director of the Government Hospital in Tel Hashomer, Sheba organized a conference in Jerusalem on the genetics of migrants and isolated populations, the first of its kind. He organized the conference because, "It had been my dream to see geneticists and hematologists from Mediterranean countries and from more remote areas assemble... in Jerusalem for a conference on environmental and inherited factors responsible for Mediterranean diseases."[39] Sheba discerned that genetics could be used as a tool for studying the issue that Maurice Fishberg and his contemporaries raised—whether the

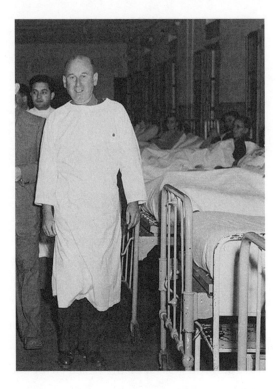

Figure 2.1. Photo of Chaim Sheba, Israeli geneticist and Director General of
the Israeli Ministry of Health. Sheba popularized the concept of
Jewish genetic diseases specific to Diaspora Jewish groups.

Jews constituted a single homogeneous group or a series of
genetically related groups.

Much had changed in the 50 years since Fishberg conducted
his studies and wrote his book on race and environment. More
than half of the Jewish population of Europe had died during
the Holocaust of World War II. Israel had been established as a
Jewish state some 13 years before. Jews from all over the world

migrated to Israel, under the Law of the Return, thus making them available as subjects for medical and scientific inquiry. The science of genetics that had been in its infancy at the turn of the century was flourishing. Genetic studies were fostered by new methods of chemical analysis for studying human variation at the molecular level. When these methods were applied to individuals with blood diseases, such as sickle cell anemia, G6PD deficiency, and hemolytic disease of the newborn, specific variants were identified that could explain their causes.

Early in his career, Sheba stumbled into human genetics in the process of preparing to practice medicine in his adopted country of Israel. Born in Bucovina, Austria, he had a religious day school (yeshiva) education that was typical for the time. He went on to study medicine at the University of Vienna, graduating in 1932. Sheba left for Palestine "with a still wet diploma, to give service to those of my friends who had left their parents' way of life in Europe and came here ahead of me, to dry the uninhabited swamps."[40] Malaria was a common disease of the swamps, not only of Palestine but throughout the coastal Mediterranean Basin. While on the boat to Palestine, Sheba read a book about tropical diseases and learned that one of the major complications of malaria was blackwater fever. Typically, in the urine of individuals with red blood cells disrupted by malarial parasites, the "black water" was the dark-colored breakdown products of the oxygen-carrying protein hemoglobin. When he arrived in Palestine, Sheba attempted to learn more about malaria by reading the local medical journal,

Harefuah. One paper by Dr. Hillel Yoffe reported the unexpected springtime occurrence of blackwater fever in 187 people, rather than the typical autumn occurrence associated with malaria. As Sheba learned, the people in Yoffe's report were not affected with malaria. Rather, they were affected with *favism,* a condition that Sheba knew about from a poem by German poet Eduard Moerike. In that poem, Moerike deplored the untimely death of his sweetheart and cursed the black and white flowers of the fava bean as the cause.[40]

Fava beans are a springtime culinary delicacy for people who live in the Mediterranean basin, yet for some individuals, exposure to the bean or even to its flowers can result in the debilitating and sometimes fatal disorder of favism.[41–42] The condition had been known in ancient Greek times. The Greek philosopher and mathematician Pythagoras is said to have warned his disciples about the dangers of eating fava beans, advice that was seconded by the philosophers Diogenes and Plutarch. The presentation and course of favism was well-characterized by Richard Lederer, another Viennese-trained physician, whose work on "Baghdad Springtime Anemia" was known to Sheba. Lederer wrote:

> The children fall ill suddenly, the start of the illness can be given by the parents as at a definite hour. Usually abdominal pains and in most cases vomiting introduce the disease. The children become conspicuously pale at once, and after a few hours jaundice starts, though the children never become as

yellow as in obstructive jaundice…In examination actually nothing is to be found besides the anaemia and the jaundice…The urine was always passed in diminished amount, concentrated and of characteristic brown colour. The analysis never showed bile pigments or bile salts, only urobilin or urobilinogen [hemoglobin pigments] in excess quantities…When recovery started, the urine very rapidly became normal.[43]

Lederer identified ingestion of beans in eight cases and merely smelling the flowers of the fava plants in another five cases! He observed that all of his patients were male, and only one was a non-Jewish Iraqi. During the 1930s, Sheba observed patients in Israel with favism. All were Jewish males of Iraqi, Yemenite, or Kurdish origin. With this discovery, he launched the idea of a heritable predisposition to favism among Jews of Middle Eastern origin.[40]

Sheba's career as a scientific investigator was derailed in the 1940s, because he served in the British Army against the Axis powers and, then, as a member of the Israeli resistance during the War of Independence against the British. Even as an Army doctor, Sheba continued his observations about hemolytic anemias—the breakdown of red blood cells leading to low cell counts. In this era, when antibiotics were first used on a wide scale, Sheba realized that severe hemolytic reactions could be provoked not only by eating fava beans but also by taking the antimalarial drugs pamaquine or primaquine or the antibiotic sulfa drugs. The reactions occurred primarily among Iraqi,

Turkish, Greek, Yemenite, and Kurdish Jewish soldiers and were also common among non-Jewish Greek and Cypriot soldiers and Italian prisoners of war. To Sheba, it was striking that the Ashkenazi Jews did not share the sensitivity to fava beans nor to primaquine that was prevalent among their co-religionists. The reason for this difference between Ashkenazi and other Jews became apparent as the genetic basis for favism and primaquine sensitivity was discovered.

Also in the 1930s, American investigators became interested in primaquine-sensitive anemia because the condition was prevalent among African-Americans, affecting up to 10% of healthy males. In 1954, Dr. Alf Alving led a team of investigators at the Army Malaria Research Unit at Stateville Penitentiary, Illinois, that identified the cause of this anemia.[44] By the time they conducted their studies, the team knew that the condition arose from a defect intrinsic in the red blood cells, preferentially affecting older red cells. Once an individual had a hemolytic reaction from exposure to primaquine or fava beans, he was immune for some weeks to a second attack until his red cells surviving the first attack had aged. The older red blood cells from these individuals had a low level of glutathione, a chemical that repaired damage to the membranes and hemoglobins of red blood cells caused by hydrogen peroxide—a process known as oxidative damage.[45] When antimalarial and sulfa drugs are being broken down in the body following ingestion, hydrogen peroxide is produced that can cause fatal damage to red blood cells if the quantity of glutathione is too low to repair the damage. (The oxidative action of hydrogen peroxide is well-known to anyone who has used a weak solution of this agent to bleach the red hemoglobin in a bloodstain.) From their knowledge of the biochemical pathway for forming glutathione, the American investigators reasoned that a defect in the enzyme glucose-6-phosphate dehydrogenase (G6PD), or another enzyme in the same biochemical pathway, could be the cause. In the course of their investigation, they showed that G6PD was deficient in the affected individuals, but that the activity of other enzymes in the pathway was normal.[44]

Arno Motulsky (Sheba's co-organizer of the 1961 Jerusalem conference and a major figure in the field of medical genetics) saw sulfa and primaquine sensitivity as part of a more general phenomenon (Figure 2.2). To account for the innate differences in the body's handling of drugs, Motulsky conceived of the concept of *pharmacogenetics*, explaining, "In discussions of drug discovery, careful distinction should be made between toxic reactions caused by immunologic mechanisms (drug allergy) and abnormal reaction caused by exaggeration or diminution of the usual effect of a given dose…Data are available now which suggest that reactions of this type may be caused by otherwise innocuous genetic traits or enzyme deficiencies."[46] People with G6PD deficiency do not get sick until they are exposed to an agent that is not toxic to other individuals. In other words, what is not toxic to the average individual is toxic to individuals with G6PD deficiency only if they are exposed to the agent. Pharmacogenetics explains not only why certain individuals

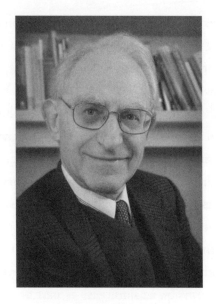

Figure 2.2. Photo of Arno Motulsky, American geneticist and one of the fathers
of medical genetics. Motulsky popularized the concept of "pharmacogenetics."

have toxic reactions to drugs but also why some individuals may
fail to respond to drugs that are effective in other people.

By the time of the conference in 1961, much was known
about G6PD deficiency.[39] Favism and primaquine sensitivity are
different manifestations of this condition. Individuals who have
had a hemolytic response to fava beans will have a similar response
when exposed to primaquine. (Subsequently, it has been shown
that the chemicals vicine and covicine, present in fava beans, are
metabolized in the intestinal tract into the strong oxidants divicine and isouramil, which can cause damage to red blood cells.[47])
The condition is transmitted as an X-linked trait (Figure 2.3).[47a]

Pattern of Transmission of an X-linked Disorder

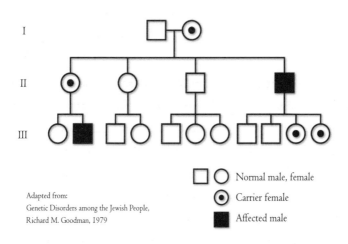

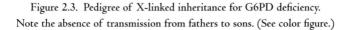

Adapted from:
Genetic Disorders among the Jewish People,
Richard M. Goodman, 1979

☐ ○ Normal male, female
◉ Carrier female
■ Affected male

Figure 2.3. Pedigree of X-linked inheritance for G6PD deficiency.
Note the absence of transmission from fathers to sons. (See color figure.)

Males have a single X-chromosome, making it more likely that
they will express the trait if their only copy of the G6PD gene
carries a mutation. The trait is never transmitted from fathers
to sons, because men transmit their Y-chromosome, rather than
their X-chromosome, to their male offspring. The gene for
G6PD deficiency is located near the X-linked genes for clotting
factor VIII and visual pigments. Individuals with mutated copies
of these genes have hemophilia and color-blindness, respectively.
In some families, the genes for two, or even three, of these conditions can be transmitted together on a single X-chromosome.
Men from these families could have color-blindness and hemophilia along with their G6PD deficiency.[48]

Females who carry mutant G6PD genes are also suscepti-
ble to hemolytic attacks if they eat fava beans or take antimalarial or sulfa drugs. Females with two copies of the mutant
gene are what Bateson termed "homozygous," which literally
means "same inheritance from eggs and sperm." (As part of
his popularization of Mendel's work, following its discovery
in 1900, Bateson coined the term "genetics," which literally
means "to give birth."[49]) Homozygous females are most susceptible to hemolytic attacks, although females with even a
single copy of the gene (the "heterozygotes" or those with
"different inheritance from egg and sperm," to quote Bateson)
may also be affected. This is explained by the presence of two
red blood cell populations in these heterozygous women: one
that has activity and one that does not. The process of ran-
domly inactivating one of the two X-chromosomes in a female
during embryonic life was described in 1961 by the English
geneticist Mary Lyon, just prior to the Jerusalem conference.[50]
This X-chromosome inactivation is stable and is transmitted
to all of the cells that are derived from the cell in which the
inactivation occurred. Lyon's observation became known as
"Lyonization" and was much commented on by the participants of the Jerusalem conference. A.C. Allison, an English
hematologist, explained the phenomenon in this way:

> There is a lot of evidence that this happens in animals.
> Several sex-linked genes giving *mottled* or *dappled* coat color in
> female mice are known — for example, "tabby." It is true also

of the tortoise-shell cat. In clones of cells in heterozygous females one finds either the full operation of the normal gene or one finds the deficient gene fully manifested, as it is over the whole body of mutant males.[39]

J.B.S. Haldane, the president of the Jerusalem conference and a founder of the field of population genetics, pointed out that Sheba showed the effects of Lyonization in his photographs of greatly magnified red blood cells. These photographs demonstrated readily discernible differences between enzyme-deficient and normal cells in heterozygous females. Other geneticists subsequently showed that the G6PD gene is subject to Lyonization in normal females.[51–52]

Although G6PD is produced and used by all of the cells of the body, only red blood cells are sensitive to the effects of oxidizing agents.[53] This occurs because mature red blood cells in circulation lack a nucleus (and therefore genetic material) that can encode the production of new enzymes. The enzyme that is produced initially has to last for the whole 120 days of a red blood cell's lifetime. Over the course of that lifetime, the amount of G6PD falls, making older red blood cells more sensitive to the oxidizing activity of fava beans and primaquine. This explains why an individual with G6PD deficiency is immune to a second attack right after a first attack. The new red blood cells have sufficient activity to ward off exposure to new oxidative damage.

Two common forms of G6PD deficiency exist: G6PD[Med] and G6PD[A-]. G6PD[Med] is prevalent across the Mediterranean basin and is found commonly among Middle Eastern and Sephardic Jews and rarely among Ashkenazi Jews. Thus, the G6PD^{Med} mutation seems to be ancient and to antedate the origins of Jewishness.[54] G6PD^{A-} is prevalent in West and Central Africa and, as a result of migration to the New World, is prevalent among African Americans and Caribbean Americans. G6PD deficiency is prevalent in regions of the world where malaria is common and may confer some protection or selective advantage to malaria. Differences in the frequency of G6PD deficiency can occur over short geographic regions if the frequency of malaria varies. The prevalence of G6PD deficiency drops off rapidly between people who live on the coast of Sardinia, where malaria is common, and people who live in the hills, where malaria is rare.[55] A similar phenomenon of high frequency along the coast and low frequency in the mountains has been observed in New Guinea.[56]

Sheba observed that the correlation of high frequency of malaria and high frequency of G6PD deficiency was not a universal phenomenon.[57] G6PD deficiency was exceptionally common among Kurdish Jews (affecting up to 70% of the male population) who lived in a mountainous region where malaria was uncommon but rare among coastal North African Jews where malaria was common.[40] Sheba was also struck that even within the same environment, the frequency of G6PD deficiency could be variable. In Iraq, G6PD was more frequent among the Jews than among their Moslem neighbors. In the Caucasus Mountains, G6PD deficiency was common among

Jews, but rare among Circassians. In Iran, G6PD was common among the Jews and Moslems, but rare among the Armenians and the Zoroastrians. From his observations, Sheba hypothesized that this variation in the frequency of G6PD deficiency reflected difference in the histories of the populations.

Over time, Sheba recognized that some diseases were found almost exclusively within certain Jewish groups, reflecting the unique history of those groups. Other conditions were shared across groups, reflecting a shared history. As Bonne-Tamir noted in her remembrance of Sheba, "But the G6PD 'story' also stimulated Dr. Sheba's thoughts in an additional direction, namely reconstruction of Jewish history and migration."[58] By 1961, it was known that Tay-Sachs disease and Gaucher disease were common among Ashkenazi Jews, familial Mediterranean fever was common among North African and Middle Eastern Jews, phenylketonuria was common among Yemenite Jews, and thalassemia was common among Kurdish Jews.[59] These diseases bore the name of the investigators who originally described them (Tay was an American ophthalmologist, Sachs was a German neurologist, and Gaucher was a French neurologist). Alternatively, the names were indicative of a biochemical abnormality (Phenylketonuria has phenylketones in the urine of affected individuals) or were descriptive of the region in which the disease was found (Thalos meant sea in Greek and like familial Mediterranean fever it was originally described in the Mediterranean basin). "Common" meant that multiple cases were described in a Jewish population that numbered in tens or hundreds of thousands. When the math is applied, the frequency of these diseases is often one in several thousand. Because most of these diseases affect only homozygotes, the disease prevalence number describes only the individuals who have two copies of the disease gene. The frequency of heterozygous individuals who carry only one copy of the disease gene was considerably higher—for example, among Ashkenazi Jews, 1:27 for Tay-Sachs disease and 1:13 for Gaucher disease.[59] Sheba assumed that these diseases were caused by transmission of a mutation that occurred sometime in the distant past and then transmitted by a group of "founders" who migrated to the Diaspora site. This phenomenon has come to be known as a "founder effect." Sheba was fond of using Biblical genealogies and spoke of conditions being transmitted by the descendents of the sons of Noah or other, later Biblical characters. As Bonne-Tamir went on to note, "His essays on these subjects were perhaps more speculation than documented facts, but they provide an excellent expression of Dr. Sheba's original reflections, his far-reaching ideas and his proficiency in Jewish and world history."[58] Thus, Sheba established the notion that these diseases served as genetic markers for the populations in which they occurred. Although not all of the members of the population carried these mutant genes, enough do to recognize a shared genetic legacy.

Although Sheba was the original force behind the concept of "Jewish genetic disease," it was Richard Goodman who had the greatest impact in popularizing this concept (Figure 2.4).[60] Goodman was an American physician who trained in medical

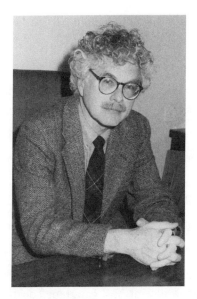

Figure 2.4. Photo of Richard Goodman, American and Israeli geneticist. Goodman wrote several influential books about Jewish genetic diseases.

genetics at Johns Hopkins School of Medicine with Victor McKusick, another of the major figures in the field of medical genetics for whom Sheba's views also had a major impact. McKusick wrote:

> One of my most cherished memories is of ward rounds with Dr. Chaim Sheba at Tel-Hashomer Hospital in 1964. As we passed from bed to bed, Dr. Sheba would say: "This is a Moroccan Jew. They are particularly susceptible to diseases A and B." Or, "This is a Yemenite Jew. They are particularly susceptible to diseases C and D." It was Dr. Sheba who stimulated my interest in the ethnic distribution of disease.[61]

McKusick published many original studies about diseases among Ashkenazi Jews, including Tay-Sachs disease and familial dysautonomia. He also compiled *Mendelian Inheritance in Man*, a catalog of all known human genetic disorders from which an Internet-based successor (*Online Mendelian Inheritance in Man*) became the standard reference in this field.[62] McKusick's example inspired Goodman to study specific genetic conditions among Jews as well as to write his own book, *Genetic Disorders among Jewish People*, which became a must-have—if not a must-read—text for geneticists, physicians, and rabbis.[63]

In 1963, Goodman went to Israel to study Buerger disease, a distinctive, painful disorder of occluded blood vessels that results in skin ulcerations, gangrene (death of tissue), and loss of fingers and toes. Most affected individuals have multiple bouts, with toes more commonly affected than fingers. Leo Buerger originally described this condition in 1908 at Mount Sinai Hospital in Fishberg's New York:

> The disease occurs frequently, although not exclusively, among Polish and Russian Jews, and it is in the dispensaries and hospitals of New York City that we find a good opportunity for studying it in its two phases, namely in the period which precedes and in that which follows the onset of gangrene. We usually find it occurring in young adults between the ages of twenty and thirty-five or forty years, and it is because of the gangrenous process may begin at an early age that the names presenile and juvenile gangrene have been employed…The

patients complain of indefinite pains in the foot, and in the calf of the leg, or in the toes, and particularly of a sense of numbness or coldness whenever the weather is unfavorable. Upon examination we see one or both feet are markedly blanched, almost cadaveric in appearance, cold to the touch...Some patients complain of rheumatic [joint] pains in the leg, others are able to walk but a short distance before the advent of paroxysmal shooting, cramp-like pains in the calf of the leg makes it imperative for them to stop short in their walk. After months or, in some cases,- even years have elapsed trophic disturbances make their appearance. It is at this stage that another rather unique symptom makes its appearance...In the pendant [hanging downward] position a bright red blush of the toes in the anterior part of the foot comes on rather rapidly, extending in some cases to the ankle or slightly above. Soon a blister, hemorrhagic bleb, or ulcer develops near the tip of one of the toes, usually the big toe, frequently under the nail, and when this condition ensues the local pain becomes intense...At the ulcerative stage, amputation may become necessary because of the intensity of the pain.[64]

Buerger's observation that most of his patients were Ashkenazi Jews would now be characterized as an "ascertainment bias"—he might have missed diagnosing the non-Jewish cases because he never saw them. Through his work with McKusick in the United States and, subsequently, with his collaborators at the government hospital in Tel Hashomer (now called "Chaim Sheba Medical Center"), Goodman determined that Buerger disease affected many different population groups, including Ashkenazi Jews. He also showed that the familial aggregation of this condition was limited, suggesting that it might not be inherited as a single-gene condition. In his book, Goodman characterized Buerger disease as a "disorder with complex or unproven inheritance," a classification that has not changed. Since Goodman's time, little progress has been made in understanding the cause of this disorder, although smoking is known to play a major role. Among Buerger's 500 cases, virtually all were smokers. Currently, the only known effective therapy to prevent amputation is complete cessation of smoking.[65] Thus, like G6PD deficiency, Buerger disease seems to be a pharmacogenetic disorder that is brought on by exposure to chemicals—in this case from cigarette smoke.

While in Israel, Goodman worked with Sheba on another study, this one about the nondisease trait of stub thumbs among various Jewish groups. Sheba believed that this condition was more common among Jews. In fact, this belief turned out to be wrong because they showed that stub thumbs were twice as common among the Israeli Arab population as among the Jewish population. Nonetheless, Goodman and Sheba's paper lent an air of excitement to this condition by noting, "This anomaly [of disproportionately short thumbs on one or both hands] has been recognized for many years and among palm readers and fortune tellers it has been called 'murderers thumbs.'"[66]

Although Goodman went back to the United States to finish his training and then to practice and teach medical genetics at The Ohio State University, the trip to Israel had a decisive impact on his life and career. In 1969, he and his family decided to return to Israel, so he could focus his career on the study and treatment of genetic disorders among Jewish peoples at Chaim Sheba Medical Center. Goodman acknowledged Sheba's influence when he wrote:

> For it was he who inspired so many of us to become interested in the genetic traits and diseases of our people. After the State of Israel came into being in 1948, waves of new immigrants from over 100 countries throughout the world came by land, sea and air to the country. They were literally met at their ports of entry by teams of physicians and geneticists, seeking to learn about the heritable differences and similarities of these people who had been dispersed for over 2000 years.[67]

Goodman went on to write his book, *Genetic Disorders among Jewish People*, because, "Through the years, as my knowledge and interest deepened concerning hereditary diseases in Jews, it became apparent that there was a need for a text to aid physicians, genetic counselors, and others who provide care for those individuals and families afflicted with these disorders."[63] Goodman's presentation was concise but comprehensive. For most disorders, he provided an historical note and then discussed clinical features, diagnosis, basic defect, genetics, prognosis and treatment, and references. To provide greater clarity, he divided the disorders into different categories for Ashkenazi, Sephardic, and Middle Eastern Jews. Recognizing that there was greater complexity than simple Mendelian inheritance patterns, he included genetic syndromes that were too rare to know whether they affected more than a few unrelated families; disorders with complex or unproven inheritance, such as Buerger disease; nondisease genetic traits, such as stub thumbs; and misconceptions about diseases. One of the misconceptions that Goodman addressed was the apparent high frequency of certain mental illnesses among Jews, a phenomenon that Fishberg had written about. Goodman wrote, "Perhaps more has been written on mental illness in Jews than on any other disorder...The older medical literature abounds with reports implying that the rate of occurrence of a variety of mental illnesses is high among Jews."[63] Goodman sought to debunk that perception by summarizing the data from two studies, one that compared the rate of hospitalization for various mental illnesses for Jews and non-Jewish European Americans in New York State and the second in Jerusalem. These studies found that the lifetime rate of psychiatric hospitalization was approximately 10.4% for the Jerusalem and New York Jews, which was slightly lower than the lifetime rate for non-Jewish European Americans. Jews who were hospitalized were more likely to have affective disorders, such as manic-depressive disease, whereas non-Jews who were hospitalized were more likely to have alcoholism (Table 2.1). Goodman concluded,

Table 2.1. Jewish and White Non-Jewish First Admissions to All Mental Hospitals in New York State, 1960–1961, Classified According to Mental Disorders.

Mental disorder	Jews Total					Non-Jews Total				
	Males	Females	No.	%	Average annual rate/100,000 pop.	Males	Females	No.	%	Average annual rate/100,000 pop.
General paresis	None	None	None	None	None	39	6	45	0.1	0.2
Alcoholic	17	2	19	0.3	0.4	1,630	464	2,094	6	8.2
With cerebral arteriosclerosis	381	521	902	16.4	18.2	3,298	3,583	6,881	19.8	26.8
Senile	178	277	455	8.3	9.2	1,266	1,941	3,207	9.2	12.5
Involutional	238	571	809	14.7	16.4	812	1,964	2,776	8	10.8
Manic-depressive	95	183	278	5	5.6	268	540	808	2.3	3.2
Schizophrenia	813	916	1,729	31.4	34.9	4,136	4,490	8,626	24.9	38.7
Psychoneuroses	246	467	713	12.9	14.4	1,676	2,644	4,320	12.5	16.9
Other	329	280	609	11	12.4	3,987	1,963	5,950	17.1	18.1
Total no. and rate	2,297	3,217	5,514	100	111.5	17,112	17,595	34,707	100	135.4

Adapted with permission from R. M. Goodman, *Genetic Disorders among Jewish People*. Baltimore: Johns Hopkins University Press, 1979.

"Thus, what once seemed certain in the minds of many – that the rate of mental illness is extremely high [in Jews]— can no longer be accepted as a truism."[63]

One of the prototypes of a Jewish genetic disease in Goodman's book was Tay-Sachs. In fact, Fishberg had made a similar distinction in his book. The disease was described in the 1880s by Warren Tay, an English ophthalmologist, and independently by Bernard Sachs, an American neurologist. For some children, Tay observed "symmetrical changes in the region of the yellow spot in each eye."[68] The reddish glow of this symmetrical change has become known as the "cherry red spot" of this condition. In his first report, Sachs observed "arrested cerebral development" and described the changes in the brain of an affected child.[69] In a follow-up study that included two other affected children from the same family, Sachs concluded that the condition was familial, associated with severe retardation, early blindness, and eventual death. To describe the condition, he coined the name, "amaurotic familial idiocy," or blind, familial, intellectual disability.[70] Almost all of these cases were Jewish. Writing about 20 years later, Fishberg noted, "At first it was thought that here an exclusively Jewish disease was at last found, because all of the cases first reported were in Jewish children." With his usual temperate point-of-view, Fishberg went on to note, "But later on many cases were described in non-Jews."[8] Indeed, many years later it was shown that Tay-Sachs disease was common among Moroccan Jews, Iraqi Jews, and also among Cajuns and French-Canadians.

By the 1970s, much was known about Tay-Sachs disease—
the appearance and clinical course, the cause, and the means for
preventing the disease. Goodman wrote:

> Infants with TSD usually appear normal at birth but by age
> 6 months parents may note that their affected child is unusu-
> ally quiet, listless, and apathetic. Early in the disease parents
> may also note difficulty in feeding and hypotonia…Some of
> these infants develop spasticity, fail to hold up their heads, and
> show abnormal limb movements. Accompanying these early
> signs is an exaggerated startle response. On hearing a sharp
> sound, infants respond with a rapid extension of both arms
> and a startled expression…By age 3 or 4 months fundiscopic
> findings [i.e., examination with an ophthalmoscope] indicate
> the development of the classic cherry-red spot…Blindness
> occurs between 12 and 18 months…Epileptiform seizures
> are common…In the terminal stage of the disease affected
> children are quiet and hypotonic and the startle reaction is
> much less exaggerated…Eventually the seizures decrease in
> frequency and severity, but progressive cachexia [wasting]
> and aspiration pneumonia usually lead to death before the
> age of 4 years.[63]

The reason for this progressive, unrelenting course was
known. Tay-Sachs falls into a class of diseases known as
"lysosomal storage disorders."[71] The lysosomes in the cell can be
compared to a garbage disposal. They contain specific enzymes
that digest the accumulated cellular garbage into small reusable

molecules. Genetic defects in the production of some of these enzymes lead to accumulation of some of these garbage molecules because alternate methods do not exist for breaking them down. In Tay-Sachs disease, the enzyme hexosaminidase A (hexA) is deficient. Ordinarily hexA would break down a fatty substance called GM2 ganglioside. Instead the GM2 ganglioside accumulates in nerve cells, causing them to balloon out and increasing their diameter two- to threefold. Over time, these nerve cells die, causing progressive neurological deterioration.

Tay-Sachs disease is inherited in an autosomal recessive manner—transmitted on a chromosome that is not a sex chromosome and requiring inheritance of two defective or mutant copies of the gene to be affected. Each of the parents of the affected children has one copy of the mutant gene and only a partial enzyme deficiency that prevents them from having the disease. Given the frequency of Tay-Sachs disease—affecting 1 in 3,600 Ashkenazi Jewish children—people in this population do not have a family history for this disorder. In the past, carriers learned of their status only after the birth of an affected child. Typically, couples with an affected child stopped having additional children because they were unwilling to face the 25% risk of Tay-Sachs disease in each subsequent pregnancy. The development of a simple, accurate, and inexpensive test that detected partial hexA deficiency in carriers and complete hexA deficiency in affected fetuses prior to birth led to the virtual prevention of Tay-Sachs disease in the Ashkenazi Jewish population by mate selection or termination of affected pregnancies.

The first program to prevent Tay-Sachs disease was initiated in the Jewish communities of Baltimore and Washington, D.C., but the concept caught on rapidly in other Jewish communities.[72] By the mid-1970s, Tay-Sachs disease screening and prevention programs existed in more than 50 U.S. cities and in other cities around the world with large Ashkenazi Jewish populations. The organization of these programs was unusual because, for the most part, testing was performed at synagogues and Jewish community centers, rather than at physician offices. Most were headed by physicians, but much of the work with outreach education, recruitment, testing, and counseling was provided by volunteers, social workers, and genetic counselors, members of a newly created profession who provided counseling and education about genetic diseases. Some programs were directed toward testing married couples, with the goal of identifying those couples in which both members were carriers of Tay-Sachs. Other carrier screening programs were aimed at university and high-school students with the goal of helping them to choose partners who were not carriers and thereby eliminating their risk for having affected children. These programs became popular among observant Jews for whom termination of affected pregnancy was not an acceptable choice.

By 1976, 151,719 people had been screened and 6,682 carriers were identified, yielding a carrier frequency of 1:23, although this figure was later revised to 1:27 when relatives of known carriers were excluded from the tally.[73] Among those screened, 124 were carrier couples. These couples were counseled about the possibility of prenatal diagnosis using amniocentesis, a newly developed procedure in which a small amount of amniotic fluid was withdrawn by needle from the sac surrounding the fetus and the cells within the fluid were tested for hexA deficiency. These couples then had the option of terminating the pregnancies of affected fetuses. The carrier couples were also counseled about the possibility of artificial insemination by non-carrier donors—an option that was not widely embraced by otherwise fertile couples. By 1996, 135 young Orthodox Jewish carriers did not make matches with other carriers.[72] As a result of these screening programs, the incidence of new cases of Tay-Sachs disease dropped by more than 90%—the few cases that occurred were among couples who had not been screened or for whom some error had been made in interpreting results. The remaining cases occurred among children who were not Ashkenazi Jewish.

The reason why Tay-Sachs disease carriers were common in the Ashkenazi Jewish population has been the subject of much speculation. Some geneticists favored natural selection as an explanation. Natural selection was the theory developed by Charles Darwin, in his treatise *On the Origin of Species* to explain why certain species thrived whereas others became extinct. He wrote:

How will the struggle for existence…act in regard to variation? Can the principle of selection, which we have seen is so potent in the hands of man [for breeding animals], apply in nature? I think we shall see that it can act most effectually…We shall best understand the probable course of natural selection by taking the case of a country undergoing some physical change, for instance, of climate. The proportional numbers of its inhabitants would almost immediately undergo a change, and some species might become extinct…We have reason to believe…that a change in the conditions of life, by specially acting on the reproductive system, causes or increases variability.[5]

So Darwin laid out two of the cardinal points of natural selection. It operated in response to some selective agent, such as climate, and the way in which it operated was to increase the reproductive fitness of some individuals so that they would have more offspring. In the case of G6PD deficiency, natural selection acted in favor of affected individuals who developed malaria. In the case of Tay-Sachs disease, natural selection acted against the affected children not surviving to adulthood to reproduce. But the selectionists presumed that the carriers of a copy of the mutant hexA gene had a selective advantage that would enable them to transmit their mutant genes and to compensate for the mutant genes not transmitted by affected children.

Among the selectionists were Ntinos Myrianthopoulos, an epidemiologist at the National Institutes of Health, and Stanley Aronson, a neurologist at Kingsbrook Jewish Medical Center in Brooklyn.[74] Regarding Tay-Sachs, they compared the number of offspring surviving to age 21 years for grandparents of children with the disease to the number of offspring for a control group of grandparents who did not have grandchildren with the disease.

They inferred for the Tay-Sachs group that one of the grand-parents had to be a carrier. They found that the carrier grand-parents had about 6% more offspring surviving to age 21 years. This exceeded the 4.5% that they calculated would be required to replace the genes that were not transmitted by the affected Tay-Sachs children. Later, Myrianthopoulos acknowledged that this sample size may not have been large enough to be certain the 6% difference had statistical significance.[75] Assuming that these grandparents had greater reproductive fitness, what was the selective agent? Drawing on the observation that tuberculo-sis (TB) was less frequent among Ashkenazi Jews than among other populations, Myrianthopoulous and Aronson suggested the Tay-Sachs carriers might be less susceptible to TB infection. The notion of resistance to infectious agents had great appeal because both G6PD and sickle cell carriers were less suscepti-ble to malaria infection. They noted that Niemann-Pick and Gaucher diseases, two other lysosomal storage diseases, were also prevalent among Ashkenazi Jews and that being a carrier for any of the three conditions might convey relative resistance to TB through a common mechanism.

The alternative explanation was genetic drift. Goodman noted:

Genetic drift can be defined as a random fluctuation in gene frequency from one generation to the next which is based on the finite size of the effective breeding population [Figure 2.5]. Thus, two generations of a population may have

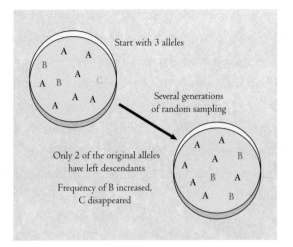

Start with 3 alleles

Several generations
of random sampling

Only 2 of the original alleles
have left descendants

Frequency of B increased,
C disappeared

Figure 2.5. Genetic drift in small populations results in random
fluctuations and increase or decrease in mutant allele frequency
from one generation to the next. (See color figure.)

different frequencies for the same gene, even though these frequencies were originally identical. Essentially the influence of
drift on gene frequency is inversely proportional to the size
of the population. For example, the chance predominance
of one genotype over another within a population will be
greater, the smaller the population.[63]

Eventually, the population would achieve a certain size
where fluctuations in the number of the affected and carrier
individuals in the next generation would have a minimal impact
on gene frequency in the whole population. At this point, the
gene frequency was said to become "fixed" in the population.[76]
Within the Ashkenazi Jewish population, which had a history

of small populations living in villages dispersed over a large geographic area, genetic drift would act to increase the frequency of some disease genes and decrease the frequency of others so that they would no longer be found within the population. Unlike selection, genetic drift did not require that these diseases have similar causes or even similar selective agents.

Drawing upon Sheba's ideas, the geneticist Victor McKusick and the epidemiologist Gary Chase proposed founder effect as an additional hypothesis for the prevalence of Tay-Sachs disease among Ashkenazi Jews.[77] Goodman defined the phenomenon in this way, "Founder effect is a special feature of drift in which some genes carried by the founders of a new community will by chance differ in frequency from those in the original, or parent, population."[63] In available geneologies, the disease mutation can sometimes be traced back to a single individual who was the "founder" in that population. For example, Queen Victoria was the founder of the hemophilia mutation that caused some of her male descendants to be bleeders, including her great-grandson, Crown Prince Alexis Nicolaievich Romanov of Russia—the Tsarevitch who was killed in the Russian Revolution.[78] In the absence of genealogies, founder effects have been inferred when the carriers for a rare genetic condition cluster seem to emanate from a particular community. Myrianthopoulos and Aronson observed that the families of Tay-Sachs carriers came from the Lithuanian and Polish provinces of Krono and Grodno (Figure 2.6). Goodman went on to observe that Ashkenazi Jewish families having children

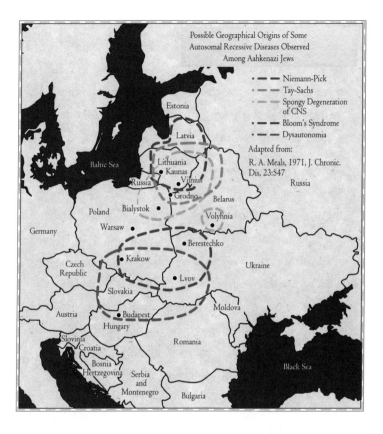

Figure 2.6. Richard Goodman's map of founder effects for common
Ashkenazi Jewish disease mutations, based on reported places of residence of
grandparents of grandparents of affected children. (See color figure.)

affected with Canavan disease, also known as "spongy degeneration of the brain," came from three areas in Eastern Europe:
the Vilna-Kovno section of Lithuania, the adjacent Bialystok
area of Poland, and the Volyhnia area of the Ukraine.[63] Most
Jewish families having children affected with Bloom syndrome

(a condition of sun-sensitive skin, severe growth retardation, and predisposition to cancer at an early age) came from the area between Warsaw and Krakow in the east and Kiev and Chernovtsy in the west, from southeastern Poland (Galicia), and from southwestern Ukraine. Goodman explained how a founder effect would work. In Goodman's words:

> These early Jewish settlements in Poland and Lithuania were composed of many small groups that often consisted of no more than a handful of families. These groups were relatively isolated genetically, not only from their gentile neighbors but also from other Jewish communities. Thus, the historical background of Ashkenazi Jewry, with its numerous small founding groups and relative genetic isolation, fits well with the features of genetic drift and founder effect and accounts for the establishment of the now characteristic Ashkenazi Jewish disease. [63]

These ideas about founder effects were proposed after World War II, so no direct sampling of gene frequencies was ever performed among pre-war Jewish residents in these Eastern European communities that would have proved a founder effect.

Other Jewish communities also had evidence for founder effects for specific diseases that arose within their communities or that arose elsewhere and were carried into the community by genetic founders. Goodman noted, "These disorders tend to be found within individual Jewish ethnic subgroups rather than dispersed among many communities that make up the two major non-Ashkenazi groups."[63] These were the disorders that Goodman catalogued and that Sheba had described to McKusick. Since the Goodman era, additional genetic conditions have been described. Currently, in different Jewish groups, almost 100 genetic conditions with Mendelian patterns of transmission are known (Table 2.2). A catalog of these conditions is maintained online (http://www.goldenhelix.org/israeli/).

Table 2.2. Genetic Conditions with Founder Mutations in Jewish Populations

Moroccan	Iranian	Ashkenazi
Tay-Sachs (not AJ)	11 beta-hydroxylase	Tay-Sachs
Corticosterone methyl	deficiency	Niemann-Pick disease
oxidase II deficiency	Hereditary inclusion body	Mucolipidosis IV
Cerebrotendinousxan-	myopathy	Gaucher disease
thomatosis	Autoimmune	Familial dysautonomia
Complement C7	polyglandular disease I	Canavan disease
deficiency	Congenital myastenia	Lipoamide dehydrogenase
Glycogen storage	gravis	deficiency
disease III	**Combined factors V and**	Glycogen storage
Factor VII deficiency	**VIII deficiency**	disease I
Ataxia telangiectasia	**Factor VII deficiency**	Maple syrup urine
BRCA1 breast and		disease
ovarian cancer	**Bukharan**	Familial hyperinsulinism
	Oculopharyngeal	Non-classical
Tunisian	muscular dystrophy	21-hyrdoxylase
Combined factors V		deficiency
and VIII deficiency	**Iraqi**	Bloom syndrome
Ataxia telangiectasia	Glanzmann thrombasthenia	Fanconi anemia
	Factor XI deficiency,	Cystic fibrosis
Libyan	**type III**	Factor XI deficiency
Cystinuria	**BRCA1 breast and**	GJB2 deafness
Creutzfeld Jacob disease	**ovarian cancer**	Usher1

(Continued)

Table 2.2. (Continued)

Habbanite	Usher3
Metachromatic	Familial Mediterranean
leukodystrophy	fever
	Idiopathic torsion
	dystonia
	Familial
	hypercholesterolemia
	BRCA 1 breast and
	ovarian cancer
	BRCA 2 breast and
	ovarian cancer
	APC Adenomatous
	polyposis coli
	Hereditary non-
	polyposis colorectal
	cancer
	Parkinson disease

Note: Conditions with shared mutations in different populations are shown in boldface.

These conditions vary in their severity and age of onset and can affect virtually any organ system. Quite strikingly, they tend to cluster into specific categories of disease (Table 2.3). Some are lysosomal storage diseases (Tay-Sachs disease, Niemann-Pick disease, Gaucher disease, and mucolipidosis IV). Some involve the accumulation of a stored form of sugar, resulting in enlargement of the liver and low blood sugar with fasting (glycogen storage diseases, types I and III). Some result in bleeding from deficiency of clotting factors (factor XI deficiency, factor VII deficiency, combined factors V and VIII deficiency). Some result in aberrant synthesis of steroid hormones that can lead to salt loss and shock or masculinization of the sex organs

Table 2.3. Genetic Disorders Among Jewish Populations Affecting Similar Biological Processes

Lysosomal storage diseases	Disorders of adrenal steroid biosynthesis
Tay-Sachs disease	21-hydroxylase deficiency
Niemann-Pick disease	11-hydroxylase deficiency
Gaucher disease	Corticosterone methyl oxidase II deficiency
Mucolipidosis IV	
Metabolic disorders	
Glycogen storage disease, I	**Disorders of DNA repair**
Glycogen storage disease III	BRCA1 breast and ovarian cancer
Lipoamide dehydrogenase deficiency	BRCA2 breast and ovarian cancer
Maple syrup urine disease	Bloom syndrome
	Fanconi anemia
Clotting factor disorders	Hereditary non-polyposis colorectal cancer
Factor XI deficiency	
Factor VII deficiency	
Combined factors V and VIII deficiency	

(21-hydroxylase deficiency, 11-hydroxylase deficiency, and corticosterone methyloxidase II deficiency). Still others result from defects in DNA repair that increase susceptibility to cancer (hereditary breast–ovarian cancer susceptibility caused by mutations in *BRCA1* or *BRCA2*, Bloom syndrome, and Fanconi anemia).[79] The reason for this clustering of diseases is not known and cannot be explained by the fact that only specialists in neurological, endocrine, and blood diseases, rather than other physician scientists, were studying Jewish populations.

The identity of these disease-causing genes, the founder mutations (usually one or two per condition) in Jewish populations, and the times at which the mutations arose within specific communities became apparent only in recent times, when new methods were developed for analyzing the DNA. This DNA analysis revealed two types of variation within the genes: the specific mutations that cause the diseases by altering the functions of the genes and the "normal variants" in the genes that generally have little impact on the genes' functions but, for the geneticist, serve as landmarks for investigating the history of these genes. Many of these normal variants arose in ancient times. As a result, these normal variants are shared across populations, providing genetic markers for common ancestry. Analysis of these markers defines the "chromosomal background" on which the specific disease-causing mutations occurred. Demonstration of a common chromosomal background for a mutation in two or more individuals indicates inheritance from the same founder.

Other, recent observations have led to the development of a method for timing when a mutation occurred, a method known as "coalescence." Coalescence is based on the observation that DNA is inherited in blocks. Sometimes a whole DNA molecule can be transmitted as an intact chromosome from one generation to the next. More commonly, the DNA is interrupted by "recombination" in an egg or a sperm cell—that is, the breakage and exchange of DNA strands between two chromosomes in a pair. The number of these recombination events measures the number of generations from a founder and determines the size of the block of DNA that has been inherited intact from him or her. Measuring the size of this block among a number of individuals who share the same mutation is one way for determining the number of generations or the coalescence to the founder. If individuals who have the same mutation share a large block, then the mutation arose in a recent founder. By contrast, if the block is short, then the founder lived a long time ago because, in each succeeding generation, part of the block has been lost by genetic recombination. Coalescence can provide a fairly precise estimate for the number of generations to the founder, in a sense, providing to genetics what carbon dating has provided to archeology and paleontology (Figures 2.7 & 2.8).

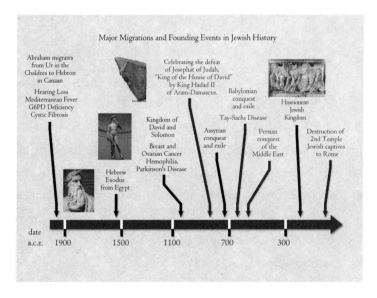

Figure 2.7. Early timeline showing coalescence of founder mutations and comparing these with events in Jewish history. (See color figure.)

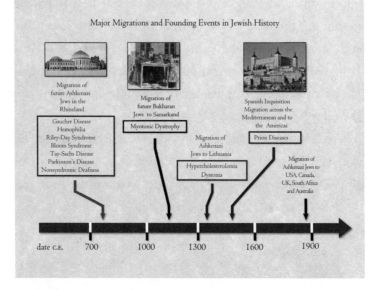

Figure 2.8. Later timeline showing coalescence of founder mutations and comparing these with events in Jewish history. (See color figure.)

By incorporating coalescence analysis along with population range of the disease, genetic conditions can be identified that were present in the ancient Mediterranean Basin, including Palestine, in pre-Jewish times. Familial Mediterranean fever represents such an example with occurrences among Ashkenazi, North African, and Middle Eastern Jews as well as Arabs, Turks, and Armenians.[80] The disease is characterized by short periodic attacks of fever and pain in the abdomen, chest, joints, or skin starting between the ages of 10 and 20 years. By coalescence theory, two mutations, called

V726A and M694V, arose more than 2,000 years ago. G6PD deficiency is another example of ancient coalescence, with its wide, Jewish and non-Jewish pan-ethnic distribution across the Mediterranean Basin.[54]

Other mutations giving rise to genetic disorders arose during the periods of Jewish rule in Palestine. Perhaps the most studied of these are the BRCA1 and BRCA2 genes, which, when mutated, give rise to breast and ovarian cancer. Often, cancer runs in families. Women with female relatives with breast and ovarian cancer are at high risk. Rosalind Franklin, the young English Orthodox Jewish scientist, who, along with Watson and Crick, discovered the structure of DNA, came from such a family—Franklin died of ovarian cancer at the age of 37 years. By its population distribution, the BRCA1 185del AG mutation is found in Ashkenazi, Iraqi, and Moroccan Jews, groups that are representative of the largest Jewish Diaspora communities. The mutation is also found among Bene Israel Jews from India and among Hispanics in northern New Mexico. Anthropologist Stanley Hordes has suggested the Hispanics from this area descended from Converso Jews who came to the New World and transmitted not only their genes but also some of their Jewish cultural practices to their contemporary, non-Jewish descendants. All of these mutations occurred on the same genetic background. This mutation is also the most common BRCA1 mutation identified among Latinos in Northern California and Spaniards in Spain.[81] A recent study from my research group supported Hordes' suggestion by showing that not only was the BRCA1 segment shared between Jews and Hispanics, but also other DNA segments, suggesting common ancestry between these groups.[81a]

Many disease mutations are unique to specific Jewish groups and are likely to have arisen in the Diaspora or to have been brought by a founder mutation carrier into the Diaspora community. The mutation may be observed to have an exclusive occurrence within a population. For example, familial dysautonomia is a disease that occurs almost exclusively among Jews with Ashkenazi Jewish ancestry. This fact serves as a criterion for diagnosis.[82] The coalescence time for a founder mutation tends to coincide with the founding of the population. Sometimes the geographic origin of the founder can be identified. Among Ashkenazi Jews, the coalescence for the common mutations in familial dysautonomia,[83] Tay-Sachs disease,[84] mucolipidosis IV,[85] Bloom syndrome,[86] factor XI deficiency,[87] Parkinson disease,[88] Usher syndrome,[89] and Gaucher disease (two mutations)[90] are approximately 40 to 50 generations ago, coinciding with the migration of Jews into the Rhineland and the founding of the Ashkenazi Jewry. Other founding events have occurred more recently. The founder mutation in the LDL receptor gene causes familial hypercholesterolemia among Ashkenazi Jews whose ancestors resided in Lithuania. The coalescence time for this mutation is 20 generations ago, which coincides with the King of Poland granting charters for Jews to reside in Lithuania.[91] The coalescence time for the common mutation in the DYT1 gene that causes the movement disorder idiopathic torsion dystonia has been calculated as 12 to 13 generations ago, which places the origin of this mutation into more recent Diaspora times in Lithuania, where this disease also arose.[84] The Gaucher disease N370S mutation was present in European populations and appears to have been introduced into the emerging Ashkenazi Jewish population.[90]

Some founder mutations coalesce to the founding of other Jewish Diaspora populations, such as the Bukharan Jews of current-day Uzbekistan. Oculopharyngeal muscular dystrophy is a disorder that is associated with weakness of the eye and swallowing muscles. It is relatively prevalent among Bukharan Jews and French Canadians, with each group having distinct founder mutations in the PABPN1 gene. The mutation in the Bukharan Jews arose 20 to 30 generations ago and coincides with the migration of Jews from Iraq to Samarkand and the establishment of this community.[92]

Mutations arose within other endogamous populations well after their founding. Among the most unusual is a heritable form of Mad Cow disease known as Creutzfeld-Jacob disease. Unlike other populations in which Creutzfeld-Jacob disease is relatively common, Libyan Jews did not consume meat from infected cows or engage in cannibalism—a practice that occurred in New Guinea where Creutzfeld-Jacob disease is also common but not heritable. Rather, the affected Libyan Jews were found to have a mutation in the PRNP prion gene, the gene that encodes the protein particle that can cause the nonheritable but transmissible form of Creutzfeld-Jacob disease. This discovery was critical for proving the role of this gene in the transmission of the disease. The coalescence time for the founder mutation in the *PRNP* gene among Libyan Jews was 23 generations ago. Twenty-three generations ago, the Libyan Jews represented the successors to the Phoenicians who settled Carthage, Helenized Jews who colonized North Africa, Jewish captives deported from Palestine to North Africa by Titus around the year 71 CE, and Berber tribes with whom the Jews engaged in cultural interactions.[93] Unlike other parts of North Africa, Libya did not serve as a major destination for Iberian Jews seeking refuge after their expulsions in 1492 and 1496. Over the last 400 years, the Libyan Jews were mostly isolated from all other Jewish populations. It is not possible to link the founding of the Creutzfeld-Jacob disease mutation to a specific historical event.

Founder mutations are sometimes shared across Jewish and gentile communities. At other times, the same mutations arose independently in several communities because they occurred at a "hotspot" of mutation. For example, the common mutation for early onset deafness is found in many population groups, including Ashkenazi Jews. This mutation was not inherited from a common ancestor who lived in the distant past. Instead, this mutation occurred many times in different groups at a region of DNA where a copying error commonly occurs and is not corrected, always with the same consequences for their offspring.[94] Although the same rare diseases may occur in Jewish Diaspora groups, they are not necessarily caused by shared founder mutations. Distinctive founder mutations arose in the HEXA gene, causing Tay-Sachs disease among Moroccan, Iraqi and Ashkenazi Jews.[95] This raises the question of whether there is something about Jewishness that gives carriers of Tay-Sachs mutations a selective advantage.

The work of the past 40 years has provided a genetic basis for Sheba's observations that Jews from different Diaspora groups had different disease susceptibilities. These observations fueled the practice of medical genetics, just as Goodman had hoped. Children with large spleens have genetic tests to determine whether they have Gaucher disease, and, in turn, receive infusions of the missing enzyme, glucocerebrosidase, replacing their depleted stores. Parents have carrier detection tests for Tay-Sachs, and a host of other disorders, to determine whether they are at risk for having affected children. Women with a strong family history of breast or ovarian cancer have *BRCA1* and *BRCA2* screening tests to define their risks for developing disease to create a personalized program of screening and prevention.

The issues of why these conditions are so common remain. Founders account for the occurrence of many of these mutations, but the prevalence of mutations must be explained by a variety of factors.[96] Genetic drift is likely to have influenced contemporary gene frequencies for all Jewish groups because many Jewish populations are known to have gone through bottlenecks as the result of wars, pograms, and disease epidemics.

Following these bottlenecks, most groups had rapid population growth that resulted from large family sizes and enhanced
survival. Among Middle Eastern and North African Jews,
consanguinity was extremely prevalent: a new mutation introduced into a family was likely to increase in frequency in future
generations.

Selection has been demonstrated to have increased the
frequency of certain conditions. Motulsky postulated and
subsequently demonstrated that carrying the gene for G6PD
deficiency conveyed resistance to malaria—that is, carriers
were less likely to develop malaria and, if infected, had milder
forms of disease with lower parasite counts.[97] This work was
built on the more familiar observation that carriers for sickle
cell disease, who had one copy of the hemoglobin S mutation,
rather than two required for being affected, were less likely to
be affected with malaria and, if infected, to have milder forms
of the disease. (The English hematologist, A.C. Allison, actually transfused Luo men in Africa with malaria-infected blood
to prove this point, an experiment that would probably be
deemed unethical today.[98]) Motulsky's observation explained
why G6PD deficiency was more common among Jews whose
families lived in recent generations around the Mediterranean
Basin, where malaria was endemic, and rare among Jews whose
families lived in Central and Eastern Europe, where malaria was
not. Natural selection for resistance to malaria also explained
Sheba's observation that G6PD deficiency was prevalent
among the Greek and Turkish soldiers and Italian prisoners of

war during World War II and why he advised the British Army against providing anti-malarial drugs to these men. Natural selection had provided the resistance to malaria that British physicians were hoping to provide with drugs.

Malaria is only one of several infectious agents that may have selected for mutations in the human genome, some of which may be deleterious. As noted, resistance to tuberculosis may have played a role and resistance to cholera may have provided an advantage to carriers of cystic fibrosis mutations.[99] Thus, natural selection is likely to have played a role in shaping the genomes of Jewish peoples. This will become a topic of active scientific investigation.

Analysis of mutations provided an indication of shared ancestry among most Jewish groups, but analysis of normal variants was needed to address the issues of lineages, bottlenecks, and genetic admixture in Jewish populations. This work on the origins and relatedness of Jewish populations started in the Sheba era. Indeed, the topic was discussed at the 1961 Jerusalem conference, but real improvement required the identification of a larger repertoire of normal variants and better methods of analysis, all of which have become available in recent years.

THREE

GENEALOGIES

Joseph Jacobs was the leading Jewish anthropologist in fin-de-siècle Europe (Figure 3.1). He was, as historian John Efron has noted, "a defender of the concept of a Jewish race."[100] He was also an historian, folklorist, and storyteller.[101–102] From an early age, Jacobs demonstrated a remarkable memory and delighted his friends with his storytelling skill. Jacobs was born in Sydney, Australia, and went to England in 1872, intending to study law and return to Australia to practice. Instead, as a student at Cambridge University, he became interested in literature and anthropology, as well as history, mathematics, and philosophy. Upon graduating in 1876, he went to London to become a writer and became immersed in the controversy about *Daniel Deronda*, a novel by the English writer George Eliot. Jacobs later

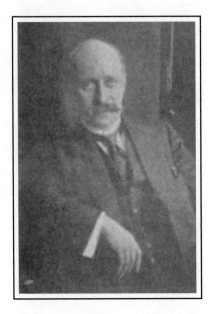

Figure 3.1. Photo of Joseph Jacobs, physical anthropologist,
polymath and Editor of the *Jewish Encyclopedia*.

recalled, "When it appeared I was just at the stage in the intellectual development of every Jew, I suppose, when he emerges
from the Ghetto, both social and intellectual, in which he was
brought up…"[103]

Daniel Deronda was Eliot's last novel and her most controversial.[104] In her earlier novels, Eliot dealt largely with pro-
vincial English life, but in her final novel, Eliot introduced
a storyline for which she was both praised and disparaged.
Daniel, the young English gentleman in search of a meaning-
ful role for his life, rescues Mirah, a young Jewish singer, from
suicide. Following this event, she disappears. As he searches

for her in London's East End, he develops an affinity for the Jewish community that resides there. In time, he discovers his own Jewish heritage, embraces Judaism, and marries Mirah.

Eliot knew of the risk that she ran writing a novel that placed Jewish culture at its center. She wrote to Harriet Beecher Stowe that she wanted "to rouse the imagination of [English] men and women to a vision of human claims in those races of their fellow men who differ from them in customs and beliefs."[105] To this end, she researched the book carefully, took Hebrew lessons, read about Jewish culture and tradition, and visited Jewish communities. Her risk-taking had the predictable effect among some of her English critics. The reviewer in the September 1876 issue of *The Academy* wrote, "We do not in the slightest degree feel 'imperfect sympathy' with Jews...the question here is whether the phase of Judaism now exhibited, the mystical enthusiasm for race, and nation, has sufficient connexion with the broad human feeling to be stuff for prose fiction to handle. We think that it has not."[105] The reviewer in the September 1876 issue of the *Saturday Review* called the Deronda storyline an "ostentatious separation from the universal instinct of Christendom." "Whether the Deronda storyline had broad appeal (I find it as appealing as Silas Marner or Middlemarch), George Eliot clearly betrayed Christendom by turning Daniel, a young English gentleman, into a Jew."[105]

Daniel's self-discovery was life-changing, not only for the character in the novel, but also for Jacobs, who, like

Daniel, found himself transformed. In the June 1877 issue of *McMillan's Magazine*, Jacobs wrote that Eliot is entitled to "the heart-deep gratitude of all Jews; the more so inasmuch as she has hazarded and at least temporarily lost success for her most elaborated production by endeavoring to battle with the commonplace and conventional ideas about Judaism" [105] Following the publication of his review, Jacobs was adopted into Eliot's circle and befriended some of the leading writers and artists of the day, including William Morris, Edward Burne-Jones, and Dante Gabriel Rossetti. Writing in *Jewish Ideals*, Joseph noted:

> George Eliot's influence on me counterbalanced that of Spinoza, by directing my attention, henceforth, to the historical development of Judaism. Spinoza envisaged for me the Jewish ideals in their static form; George Eliot transferred my attention to them in their dynamic development. Henceforth I turned to Jewish history as the key to the Jewish problem.[103]

Elliot not only galvanized Jacobs to study Jewish history, but her novels provided him with a framework for his observations. He wrote, "It is difficult for those who have not lived through it to understand the influence that George Elliot had upon those of us who came to our intellectual majority in the Seventies. George Elliot's novels were regarded by us not so much as novels, but rather as applications of Darwinism to life and art."[103]

To learn about Jewish history and texts, Jacobs went to Berlin in 1877 to study with the distinguished Jewish scholars

Moritz Steinschneider and Moritz Lazarus. As John Efron has noted in his book, *Defenders of the Race*:

> Jacobs' view of Jewish history was integral to his anthropological writings on the Jews...He was convinced that certain races and nations were unique, and that these racial differences, which revealed themselves in the intellectual output of a race, were decisive. Jacobs felt that a study of Jewish history, when combined with an analysis of Jewish racial characteristics, would provide him with a powerful arsenal in the battle against the anti-Semites and therefore with a possible solution to the Jewish question. He regarded it as his duty to fight anti-Semites of his day by pointing out Jewish "contributions to civilization."[100]

To learn about Darwinism upon his return to England, Jacobs apprenticed himself to Charles Darwin's cousin, Francis Galton, himself a famous polymath. As visitors to the Galton Museum at University College in London observe today, Galton believed that all human attributes could be measured—heads, heights, intelligence. In his presidential address to the Anthropology Section of the British Association for the Advancement of Science in 1885, Galton stated, "The object of the Anthropologist is plain. He seeks to learn what Mankind are in body and mind, how they came to be what they are, and whither their races are tending; but the methods by which this definite inquiry has to be pursued are extremely diverse."[106] Jacobs applied Galton's methods to measuring Jews and wrote

Jewish Statistics: Social, Vital and Anthropometric.[22] Unlike his friend, Maurice Fishberg, Jacobs concluded that the low historical rates of intermarriage and proselytism and the physical resemblance among Jews favored the idea of a Jewish race. In his article in the *Jewish Encyclopedia* on "Anthropology," he wrote, "The remarkable unity of resemblance among Jews, even in different climes, seems to imply a common descent."[20]

Jacobs made a prediction that would be tested nearly a century later. He wrote, "One branch of Jews, the Cohanim, are prevented by Jewish law from marrying even proselytes, and yet the Cohens do not appear to differ anthropologically from the rest of Jews. This might be used to prove either the purity of the race or the general impurity of the Cohens."[22]

This notion of exploring the deep ancestry of one group of Jews was picked up in 1997 by a team of anthropologists and geneticists from the United Kingdom, Israel, and the United States who identified a set of genetic markers that at first pass seemed to be characteristic of Cohanim and, by extension, of Jewishness.[107] In turn, this study of the deep ancestry of Cohanim has led to similar studies of many Jewish groups.[108]

Jewish identity has maternal and paternal strands. Since Talmudic times, Jewish identity has been acquired through the maternal line or by rabbinically authorized conversion. Yet within the Jewish community, membership in the three male castes—Cohan, Levite, and Israelite—is acquired through the paternal line—Cohan fathers have Cohan sons. This tradition has been transmitted orally and with surnames: Cohanim (plural for Cohan) are commonly called Cohen, and Levites are commonly called Levy. Jews that are neither Cohanim nor Levites are Israelites. These castes have existed since Biblical times. The first Cohen was Aaron, the brother of Moses. Both Aaron and Moses were members of the tribe of Levi, the descendants of the third son of the patriarch, Jacob. Levi, the smallest of the 12 tribes, was designated as having priestly status, replacing the prior practice of the priestly class being comprised of firstborn sons (Numbers 3:12).

In ancient times, the Cohanim officiated in the Temple, the center of Jewish religious life.[109] They oversaw sacrifices and other Temple-based rituals and served as lawgivers, legal scholars, and magistrates of criminal and civil disputes. The priesthood survived the Babylonian exile and enjoyed both religious and secular leadership during the Hasmonean times. It was only during Roman times that the power of the priesthood waned and was replaced by rabbinical religious leadership. Nevertheless Cohanim have retained religious status. In the synagogue, they are first to be called to read the Torah. They are exempt from paying a special tax on the birth of a firstborn male. They are forbidden entry into a cemetery or, as noted, from marrying a convert. In some Jewish communities, Cohan status is recorded on grave headstones, which has provided an unofficial census for membership in these groups. From counting the number of headstones in two London cemeteries, the English geneticist Neil Bradman estimated that Cohanim comprise about 4% of the Jewish people.[110] So Cohanim is part of an orally and genetically transmitted tradition, but are all Cohanim descendents of the tribe of Levi?

In the 1990s, genetic testing became available to examine lineages and origins. Through the work of the population geneticists Michael Hammer, Luca Cavalli-Sforza, and others, genetic testing of the Y-chromosome could establish and trace male lineages.[111–112] In recent times, this has become quite precise.[113] Y-chromosomes are comprised of 60 million bases of DNA that encodes genes that cause the bearer to become a male and to transmit his Y-chromosome and other genes to his offspring. Y-chromosomal DNA is transmitted stably from one generation to the next, but minor variations occur along the way. Some of the variants have occurred only once during human history, whereas others occur as frequently as once in every 500 transmissions. These variants have occurred in different places at different times. These variants marked the Y-chromosomes of men who once lived in a certain region of the world and whose contemporary relatives might still live there or have been dispersed to another place. The patterns of Y-chromosomal variants (called Y-chromosomal types or haplotypes or haplogroups) among contemporary men distinguish male lineages.

These Y-chromosomal haplotypes are named by a capital letter followed by a string of letters and numbers—these designations are subject to revision every few years as new discoveries are made.[113] The E3b lineage (since renamed E1b1b, by a volunteer naming group, called the Y Chromosome Consortium) was found among all of the Ostrer males. It arose about 20,000 years ago in a Middle Eastern man whose descendants were among the first farmers who helped to disseminate agriculture in the Middle East.[114] Men who carried this Y-chromosome brought agriculture into Europe, North Africa, and the Horn of Africa. As a result, this Y-chromosomal pattern is common among men who live in those regions today. It was also present in men who chose a Jewish way of life; thus, it is common today among Ashkenazim and other Jews—Syrian, Kurdish, Djerban, and Yemenite Jews. It demonstrates that these Jews are the descendants of people who once lived in the Middle East.

How do we know that E3b male ancestor lived 20,000 years ago? Because they are known to occur with a fairly fixed rate, the variants on the Y-chromosome variants provide a molecular clock for timing events in human history that can be measured in generations. Each insertion, deletion, or substitution of DNA in the sequence of the Y-chromosome represents a tick of the molecular clock (Figure 3.2). Comparison of the Y-chromosomes of two individuals or of multiple individuals in a group will lead to the time of the most recent common ancestor, usually measured as a number of generations. According to the clock devised by the geneticist Bruce Walsh, for individuals whose Y-chromosomes are identical at 37 different sites, the time to a common ancestor is 5 generations.[115] If there is a mismatch at one of those sites, then the time to a common ancestor is 12 generations; and if there are two mismatches, then the time to a common ancestor

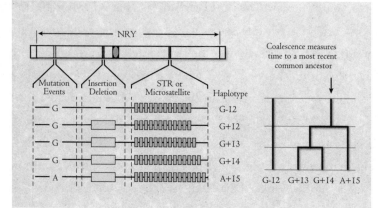

Figure 3.2. The combination of markers genotyped at polymorphic sites
anywhere on the Y-chromosome of each male is referred to as a haplotype.
Coalescence of the various markers measures the time to a
most recent common ancestor. (See color figure.)

is 19 generations. Several Y-chromosomal molecular clocks have
been applied to men from geographically dispersed populations
to time the occurrence of a common male ancestor, a "Molecular
Adam," whose Y-chromosome is more similar to ours than to our
great ape ancestors. According to this clock, Molecular Adam
lived in Africa 125,000 years ago and, by chance alone, transmitted his Y-chromosome to the ancestors of contemporary humans.
As humans originated 150,000 to 200,000 years ago, Molecular
Adam was not the first man and other men were likely to have
lived in Molecular Adam's time. Rather, Molecular Adam was
the lucky male who was able to transmit his Y-chromosome to
future generations of men around the world.

Y-chromosomal analysis has shown that most Diaspora Jews whose ancestors lived only one or two generations ago in Europe, North Africa, or the Middle East were descended from a smaller group of men who once lived in the Middle East.[116] Muslim and Christian men who live in the Middle East today have similar lineages and were descended from some of the same ancestors. These Y-chromosomal lineages define contemporary Semitic populations, all descended from Molecular Adam but apparently not all descended from an ancestral "Noah" or even from an ancestral "Abraham." Among contemporary Ashkenazi Jews, seven different Y-chromosomal lineages (E3b, G, JI, J2, Q, R1aI, and R1b) are common, accounting for more than 80% of the total (Figure 3.3).[117] Of these, five Y-chromosomal lineages (E3b, G, JI, J2, Q) were part of the ancestral gene pool transmitted by Jews who migrated from the Middle East, and at least two (R1aI and R1b) entered the Ashkenazi Jewish population after their dispersal to Europe. Yet this distinction of European/Middle Eastern in the Ashkenazi gene pool may not be quite so simple. During the Stone and Bronze Ages, Europe was colonized by settlers from the Middle East, who brought agriculture, horses, bronze, and chromosomes with them, so that some of these Middle Eastern Y-chromosomal lineages were brought to Europe during those early times then introduced through admixture between Europeans and Jews, whereas other lineages were brought to Europe by the Jewish ancestors of Ashkenazim.[118]

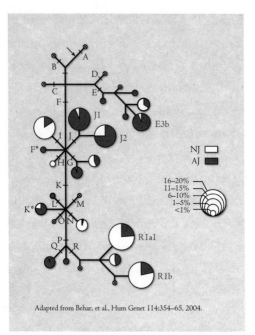

Adapted from Behar, et al., Hum Genet 114:354–65, 2004.

Figure 3.3. Y-chromosomal haplogroups among Ashkenazi Jews
demonstrate descent from a discrete set of founders. (See color figure.)

All seven common Y-chromosomal lineages might represent
founder events in the Ashkenazi Jewish population—that is,
Ashkenazi Jews may be descended from seven families, each
of which had its own Y-chromosomal lineage.[117] Comparing
the frequency of these lineages among contemporary Jews to
European non-Jews has led to an estimate of an overall historical rate of 5% to 8% admixture or intermarriage with
European populations since the founding of the population.

This is equivalent to a rate of admixture of 0.5% per generation and contrasts sharply with the 30% to 50% rates of admixture that have occurred in recent generations.[116] The presence of these European Y-chromosomal lineages is the major difference between Ashkenazi and Middle Eastern and Sephardic Jews.[119] The Y-chromosomal analyses provide evidence of founder events, both from the migration of people whose origin was in the Middle East and from Eastern European people who mixed with the Ashkenazi Jewish population—akin to what has been observed with founder disease mutations.[120]

The ancestral lineages of the J1 and J2 Ashkenazi Jewish Y-chromosomal haplogroups are also illustrative of the history of the populations from which Ashkenazi Jews were derived.[114] Along with E3b, J1 and J2 are the most common Y-chromosomal types among Ashkenazi Jews. J1 and J2 arose in the ancient Middle East from a parental Y-chromosomal type called J. Given its current distribution, J1 may have arisen in present-day Israel or southern Mesopotamia. It is common not only among Ashkenazi and Sephardic Jewish men but also among Bedouin tribes and Arabic speakers of Syria, Iraq, the Sinai Peninsula, and the Arabian Peninsula. It was spread by Semitic language speakers to northern Africa, where it is prevalent among the Arabic speakers of Algeria, and to Ethiopia, where it is prevalent among the Amhara, the speakers of a Semitic language. The frequency of Haplogroup J1 drops off at the borders between Arabic countries and non-Arabic countries, such as Turkey and Iran. Haplogroup J1 is frequent among certain populations in the northeast Caucasian region of Dagestan, representing a founder event there. Haplotype J1 was transmitted to small numbers of men residing in contemporary Sicily, southern Italy, Spain, Azerbaijan, Turkey, and Pakistan, most likely by Arabs and Phoenicians traders and conquerors or by Jewish traders.

Haplogroup J2 is thought to have originated in the Anatolia region of Turkey or in northern Mesopotamia (the region from which Patriarch Abraham came) and to have spread with the migrations of Bronze Age Anatolian farmers to other parts of the Middle East, Europe, Central Asia, and South Asia. J2 is found commonly among Turks, Muslim Kurds, Georgians, Iranians, Iraqis, Tajik and Pakistanis, and among the men of western and southwestern India, representing the Aryan migration into the Indian subcontinent. Its frequency drops rapidly in the Carpathian basin and in Afghanistan.

Yet as noted, not all of Ashkenazi Jewish male origins can be related to the migration of Jewish men from the Middle East. After E3b, J1, and J2, the most common Ashkenazi Jewish Y-chromosomal types are R1a1 and R1b, with frequencies of 7.5% and 10%, respectively.[117] R1a1 is very common among Ukrainians (where it is thought to have originated), Russians, and Sorbs (Slavic speakers in Germany), as well as among Central Asian populations. This may, in fact, be the signal of the admixture of Khazars with Ashkenazi Jews, although the admixture may have occurred with Ukrainians, Poles, or Russians.[120] R1b is the most common Y-chromosomal type of Atlantic Europe with very high frequencies among the Welsh, Basques, Irish, English, Portuguese, French, and Dutch. Its occurrence among Ashkenazi Jews may be an indicator of admixture that occurred at the time of Jewish residence in the Rhine Valley prior to the migration to Eastern Europe.[120] This haplogroup is also prevalent among the Marronite Christian community in Lebanon and represents the establishment of a European enclave in Lebanon by religious Crusaders in the eleventh to thirteenth centuries C.E.[121]

So what of the Cohanim? Karl Skorecki, a Canadian-born nephrologist and geneticist, conceived of such a study while he was praying in his synagogue near his home in Haifa, Israel. Skorecki told the journalist Jon Entine, "I was interested in the question: To what extent was our shared oral tradition matched by other evidence?"[122] Using two Y-chromosomal markers, Skorecki and Michael Hammer identified a Y-chromosomal type that was more prevalent among Ashkenazi and Sephardic Cohanim than Israelites.[107] Subsequently, Thomas, Bradman, and Goldstein added more genetic markers, for a total of six.[108] The pattern commonly observed about Cohanim males was referred to as the Cohanim Modal Haplotype (CMH). It was called a modal haplotype, because many Cohanim males diverged at one or more markers, usually by 1 unit of that marker. Goldstein calculated the time to a most recent common male ancestor and determined that the Cohanim Y-chromosomal lineage arose 106 generations ago. If the generation time is 25 to 30 years, then the progenitor of this Y-chromosome lived 2,650 to 3,180 years ago, suggesting that the founding of the lineage occurred during the Temple period.[108] This finding generated considerable excitement, because it was taken as evidence of the fidelity of an oral tradition extending over millennia. In his book, *Jacob's Legacy*, Goldstein said that he felt "like a window had opened from the modern world into something ancient, powerful and hidden…Our results appeared to be a striking confirmation of the oral tradition."[123] The CMH became an informative marker of ancestry that could be used to test for membership in this caste. "The men walk a little taller after learning that they are Cohanim, members of the priestly caste," Neil Bradman told me, "Even the scientists!"

Over time, the excitement about the CMH results has been tempered by other observations. Scozzari and her coworkers have written somewhat disparagingly, "Earlier work based on fewer Y-chromosome markers led to rather simple historical interpretations and highlights the fact that many population-genetic analyses are not robust to a poorly resolved phylogeny."[124] When applied to the CMH, it has been discovered this Y-chromosomal set of markers is not unique to Jewish men.[125] It is found commonly among other Middle Eastern men, including those in Yemen, Oman, Iraq, and Palestine, where frequently 20% or more of the male population has Y-chromosomes with this haplotype. Analysis of additional genetic markers (unique event polymorphisms, rather than microsatellite markers) has shown that the CMH occurs on two different ancestral Y-chromosomal types—JI and J2—with roughly half occurring on each.[126] These two haplogroups diverged from each other about 25,000 years ago. Among men with the CMH and the J1 haplogroup, the time to a most recent common ancestor was 8,700 years ago, whereas among men with the J2 haplogroup, the time to a most recent common male ancestor was 17,900 years ago. Entine has put forth the idea that these two CMHs reflect dual origins of Jewish priests—Aaronite and the Zadokite. Zadok functioned as a priest during the time of Kings David and Solomon.[122] His sons continued their priesthood up to the time of the Babylonian exile. Zadok may or may not have been a descendant of Aaron. Entine's speculation exceeds what can be supported by the current genetic record. Nonetheless, this record refutes the idea of a single founder for Jewish Cohanim who lived in Biblical times. The investigators at the Sorenson Molecular Genealogy Foundation who made these observations have warned, "The inference of Jewish ancestry based on the original CMH definition should be performed with caution as subjects may be falsely categorized into the eponymous CMH lineage when the true origin is in the deeply divergent…branch."[125] In essence, they are warning consumers of genetic tests to beware.

Nonetheless, these results still supported the notion of common origins of CMH lineages in the Middle East, before the Diasporas of the Jewish people into separate communities. They also supported the notion that the majority of contemporary Jewish priests descended from a limited number of male founders. The CMH on the most common J1 haplogroup was redefined by 12 microsatellite markers ("extended CMH") and another genetic marker that is prevalent in the Middle East. This lineage has been found among 46% of Cohanim, both Ashkenazi and non-Ashkenazi, and is absent among non-Jews. In Hammer and Skorecki's estimate, the coalescence time for this lineage was 3,190—not remarkably different from what was reported originally. The J2 Cohanim lineage was found among 14.4% of Ashkenazi and non-Ashkenazi Cohanim and was estimated to have arisen 4,415 years ago.

Using observation about the prevalence of the CMH, the British anthropologist Tudor Parfitt and his collaborators startled the world with their observation that members of a Black African tribe, known as the Lemba, were the descendants of Jews. In an article published in 2000 entitled "Y Chromosomes Traveling South: The Cohen Modal Haplotype and the Origins of the Lemba—the 'Black Jews of Southern Africa,'" Parfitt and coworkers believed they provided evidence for the Lemba's claim of Jewish ancestry.[127] The work was popularized in the press and in a NOVA television series so that the Lemba joined the popular conception of Jewish genetics, along with Cohan Y-chromosomes (which some of Lemba have), Tay-Sachs disease, and susceptibility to breast cancer.[128]

The Lemba have certain practices that mirrored those of the Jews—not eating pork and the ritual slaughter of animals. According to their legends, they were descended from ancient tribes in Judea who migrated to southern Africa via a place called Sena (which may be Sanaa in modern Yemen).

In southern Africa, they believed that they built an ancient civilization called Great Zimbabwe before moving on to other parts of Africa. Zimbabwe ("great house of stone") is the largest ancient ruin in sub-Saharan Africa. Parfitt has stated that at first he did not believe the Lemba's claim of Jewish identity.[129] These beliefs might have been imposed by missionaries, so he and his coworkers decided to test the hypothesis of Jewish ancestry by determining whether the CMH was also present among a significant proportion of their Lemba. Their study found the presence of this Y-chromosomal type among a high proportion of Lemba men, including 50% of men in the Buba subtribe. As noted, the CMH is found among Semitic people other than Jews so the study points to Semitic, albeit not necessarily Jewish, origins among the Lemba. Their ritual practices might be of Islamic, rather than Jewish, origin. And as noted, the CMH is not a unique marker of Jewishness.

The study of Y-chromosomes among the Levites also yielded unexpected surprises.[130] The Levites were the priestly helpers—never accorded all of the rights and responsibilities of the Cohanim. In Temple times, the Levites were responsible for the upkeep of the Temple, transporting the Ark of the Covenant, and reading second from the Torah. Over time, their responsibilities grew to include teaching, administration, and interpretation of Jewish law and ritual, as well as the composition and performance of liturgical music. These functions became important during the Hellenistic period and led Jewish worship away from the Temple and into synagogues and home.

Like Cohanim, today, Levites account for about 4% of the Ashkenazi male community and somewhat less in the Sephardic communities.[110]

Y-chromosomal analysis of Levites has demonstrated multiple origins that depend on the Diaspora community from which they came—they are not all the descendants of tribal founder Levi. Using the same methods applied to Cohanim, the Sephardic Jews from Diaspora communities in North Africa and the Middle East were found to have the CMH as their most common lineage, comprising about one-third of the Levite Y lineages. (Some have argued that this figure is as high as 51%.) Two other Levite Y-chromosomal lineages are also common among Ashkenazi and Sephardic Israelites. These findings were interpreted as showing that the Sephardic Levites are not merely the descendents of members of the tribe of Levi but also have had significant influx from among Israelites.

The findings among the Ashkenazi Levites were quite different from those among Sephardic Levites. About 10% of Ashkenazi Levites had the CMH, and 50% had the R1a1 haplogroup—a Y-chromosomal lineage of Eastern European, non-Jewish origin. As noted, this lineage is found at high frequency among Ashkenazi Jewish Israelites, as well as the Slavic-speaking Sorbians, Belarussians, Poles, Russians, and Ukrainians. Using the molecular clock-timing mechanism for this major lineage among the Ashkenazi Levites, the time to a most recent common male ancestor was approximately 1000 years ago—around the time that Ashkenazi Jews were populating Eastern Europe and possibly around the time that the Khazars were converting to Judaism. Whether this founder Levite and his brothers and sons converted to Judaism or were the descendents of European or Central Asian people long converted to Judaism is unknown. Their descendents then went on to populate the Ashkenazi Jewish communities around Eastern Europe. Nonetheless, this observation may be undermining the status of Ashkenazi Levites. One approach that Jewish legal scholars have taken toward Y-chromosomal origins is "majority rule." If the majority of Levites in a community appear to have shared origin, then all within that community are assumed to have that origin. If the majority of Ashkenazi Levites had a European or Asian male founder, then they must not be the descendents of a Biblical Levite. These observations demonstrate how identification of the historical record through the use of genetics, albeit imperfect, can create potential divisions or perceptions of illegitimacy within a community. Skorecki, the co-discoverer of the CMH, disagreed with this notion of majority rule by noting, "Talmudic law states that we should accept at face value the word of one who claims that they are of the priesthood"[122] In his original research paper, Skorecki wrote:

> This may be because there are more rights and duties associated with the Cohen status than with that of the Levite, leading to more rigorous protection of the former...Indeed,

Talmudic sources may possibly be interpreted to support the notion of differences in the social, religious, and legal barriers that relate to the assumption of Cohen and Levite status.[130]

He then went on to describe how this might happen based on "a Talmudic passage describing a debate regarding the potential assignment of Levite status to a man (and his descendants) whose father was a non-Jew and whose mother was the daughter of a Levite. Such differences could have provided the backdrop for the sanctioned acceptance of Levite status other than through patrilineal descent."

Linguistics might also shed some insight into the origins of some Ashkenazi Jews. Geneticists Luca Cavalli-Sforza, Paolo Menozzi, and Alberto Piazza have observed that people who speak the same language tend to share the same genes. They have demonstrated that genetic boundaries, defined as regions of rapid genetic change, tend to coincide with linguistic boundaries. They have written, "It is unlikely that a sharp boundary in a continuously inhabited region is due to change in natural selection across the boundary; it is more likely that it signals a local decrease in genetic exchange."[131] They go on to note, "Local decrease could be due to one or more of a great variety of barriers limiting exchange between two regions. The first and most natural are geographic boundaries: the sea, mountains and major rivers.... Language differences are also high on the list of expected barriers."

Jewish dialects of local languages arose during the Jewish Diasporas. Judeo-Spanish (Ladino), Judeo-Persian, Judeo-Arabic, and Judeo-German (Yiddish) were all local languages to which Hebrew or local vernacular Jewish words were added. During a visit to Congregation Ezra Bessaroth in Seattle, a Sephardic Jewish synagogue that was established by Sephardic Jews from Turkey and the Island of Rhodes, I heard the Latino language used during the service. It was recognizable, if not completely comprehensible, as a dialect of Spanish that developed following the Spanish Inquisition among the Jews who migrated to the Ottoman Empire. It is still used today among the descendants of these Jews who live in Turkey, Serbia, Bosnia, Bulgaria, Israel, and Greece, although not commonly.[132] Ladino is most similar to Castilian Spanish of the fifteenth century but contains many old Hebrew and Talmudic words. Some of the Castilian words have entirely disappeared from the vocabulary of modern Spanish or are rarely used now. At Congregation Ezra Bessaroth, the aliyot (the honors of reciting prayers over the reading of the Torah) are auctioned off. My host bid so that I would have the honor of the first aliyah. The bidding got intense as it reached *trenta mil* (30,000) pennies!

The prevailing view has been that Ashkenazi Jews acquired the Yiddish language as a dialect of German when they lived in the Rhineland region, then brought this language with them to Eastern Europe. In Eastern Europe, Yiddish became a Creole language in which Hebrew and Slavic words were incorporated, a process known as "relexification."[133] Yiddish is not a uniform language; rather, it is a generic name for a number of dialects that differ considerably from one another, of which three groups are recognized—the southern dialect that was spoken in Rumania and the south of Russia, the Polish dialect, and the Lithuanian dialect. These dialects are sufficiently intelligible to one another, just as Bavarians, Silesians, and Alsatians can understand each others' dialects of German.

Paul Wexler, a linguist at Tel Aviv University, has turned this theory on its head by suggesting that based on its grammar and idioms, Yiddish was of Slavic origin and then relexified with German words and written with Hebrew characters.[134] He has speculated that these relexification events occurred twice, once in the Upper Sorbian Slavic-speaking region of Germany and a second time in the Kiev-Polessian Slavic-speaking region of contemporary Ukraine and Belarus, and that these separate events account for the dialectic differences. According to Wexler's theory, the Yiddish language would represent a marker for the admixture that occurred between Eastern European Slavic speakers and Jews migrating from Germany. The fact that Ashkenazi Jews spoke Yiddish and their neighbors spoke a variety of different Slavic, Germanic, or other languages probably contributed to the genetic isolation of the Jews. Yiddish may then have acted as a genetic isolating mechanism, although the proscriptions on intermarriage and proselytism may have had an equally profound effect.

So what about the other famous Jewish lineage that was established by King David? David and his son, Solomon, were the great kings of Israel. During his 33-year reign, David established Israel as a united and regional power. David is famed not only for his military, civil, and religious accomplishments but also for the prophecy that the Messiah would come from his lineage—Christians believe that Jesus Christ was the Messiah and a descendent of King David. Although some have deemed King David to be a mythical figure, the identification in 1991 of a stone in the town of Tel Dan, Israel provided evidence for the House of David in the archeological record. This stone Jerusal has become known as the "House of David Inscription" and is deemed to provide proof of the Davidic lineage.[136]

David's lineage continued after his death. Following the division of the Kingdom of Israel, members of the House of David continued to rule the Kingdom of Judah up to the time of the Babylonian exile in 586 B.C.E. Jehoichin, the last King of Judah, moved with his people to Babylon and became the Exilarch, or Prince of Captivity. The Exilarch was a hereditary office that carried both religious and civil authority. With the exception of a period in the sixth century C.E. when the office was abolished following a revolt, this position existed for more than 1,500 years and survived changes of rule in Babylon.[31] The last Exilarch moved from Babylon to Spain in the twelfth century, and it is from him that claims of linkage to the Davidic lineage are made. Both Moshe Shaltiel Gracian and Arthur Menton developed extensive genealogies that linked their male relatives to the Exilarch. Menton has described the result of his research on the Charlap lineage in *The Book of Destiny*,[137] and Shaltiel Gracian has described his genealogy of the Shaltiels and Gracians on his website, Shaltiel.com.[138] Much like the Cohanim and Levites, if there were a traceable Davidic lineage, then it would be found among a significant fraction of men who claimed descent. Bradman and his co-workers performed the analysis for the members of the Shaltiel, Gracian, and Charlap families. The findings showed that the Y-chromosomal lineages followed the surnames of the men who participated but that there was no linkage across surnames. As Bradman noted, there may be a Davidic lineage, but it is hard to know who carries it based on the results of this project. So why did the search for a Davidic Y-chromosomal lineage flop? Despite the best efforts, genealogies are incomplete. Within those lineages, paternity is not always stated correctly. Children are adopted, and although the father's surname is taken, the adoption may not be recorded.

This work has highlighted that genetic testing has become an important tool for genealogists. They have taken advantage of the commercial genetic testing services to establish their own Y-chromosomal lineages, to link them to their surnames, and to test their own hypotheses of shared ancestors with like-named men. Some men will walk taller when they learn about shared ancestry with the Cohanim. Others will be surprised to learn about their ancestral skeletons in the closet.

Shaltiel Gracian is a dedicated genealogist who hopes that with more work, a Davidic Y-chromosomal lineage will be discerned, but for the time being, it is impossible to validate the claims of any of the aspirants.

Much similar work has also been done on maternal lineages. In fact, prior to the identification of Molecular Adam, there was Mitochondrial Eve. Mitochondrial Eve was identified by Rebecca Cann and Allan Wilson by studying mitochondrial DNA.[139] The mitochondria are small organelles in the cells that convert fats and carbohydrates into a form of energy that the rest of the cell can use. The mitochondria contain small, circular molecules of DNA that encode some of the genes that play a role in this energy utilization. Mitochondria and, by extension, mitochondrial DNA are transmitted by mothers through egg cells to offspring (Figure 3.4). Thus,

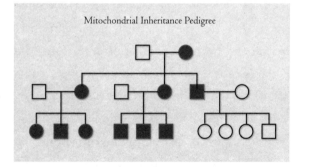

Figure 3.4. Pedigree of mitochondrial inheritance demonstrating maternal transmission to offspring. (See color figure.)

mitochondria DNA shows a pattern of maternal transmission and provides a way for looking at matrilineal inheritance. Cann and Wilson argued that if they looked at the mitochondrial genomes of many women, they would be able to apply coalescence theory and identify the mother of our mitochondrial genomes (or at least the time to a most common recent ancestor in the form of)—a Mitochondrial Eve. Like their successors, they argued that "molecular clocks stemmed from the observation that rates of genetic change from point mutations (changes in individual DNA base pairs) were so steady over long periods that one could use them to time divergences from a common stock."[140] Their investigations demonstrated that Mitochondrial Eve lived in Africa some 175,000 years ago. So if Mitochondrial Eve and Molecular Adam were not contemporaneous, how could they have gotten together and given rise to contemporary humans?

Coalescence theory identifies the most recent common ancestors but does not presume that other reproductive individuals were absent from the population at the time of that progenitor—the effective population size is thought to have been around 10,000 in the era of Mitochondrial Eve. Rather, coalescence theory identifies the ancestor who by reproductive prowess, selective advantage, or chance had his or her line transmitted to many subsequent generations. Could others have had similar reproductive success that left a genetic signature in our genomes? Reich and his colleagues provided evidence for so-called "rehybridization" events between early hominids and chimpanzees by analyzing the sequence of human X-chromosomes with those of chimpanzees. They explain their results in this way, "These unexpected features would be explained if the human and chimpanzee lineages initially diverged, then later exchanged genes before separating permanently."[141] Rehybridization is not the norm. Based on their analysis of the human X-chromosome, Hammer and his colleagues have provided evidence that early humans may have lived for extended periods of time in relatively isolated groups, followed only recently by interbreeding.[142] Thus, human evolution has not been a straight path from chimpanzees to Adam and Eve to the present.

Analysis of Jewish mitochondrial genomes in some Diaspora communities has demonstrated limited genetic diversity and, therefore, strong founder effects. Behar and his coworkers found four common types of mitochondrial genomes (called "haplogroups" among geneticists) accounting for 70% of the total among Ashkenazi Jews, suggesting four founder females for the populations (Figure 3.5).[143] Based on comparison with non-Jewish populations of different geographic origins, several of these founders originated in the Middle East and their descendants migrated to Eastern Europe by way of the Rhineland. Other founders originated in Europe; thus, these findings are similar to what has been observed for Ashkenazi Jewish male founders. Evidence for founder females has been observed in other Jewish populations, although the number of founders and the relative proportion of founders from one population to another is variable.[144]

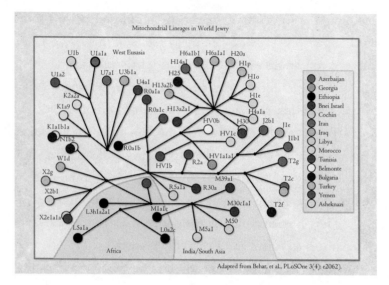

Figure 3.5. Mitochondrial lineages among World Jewry and geographical
locales from which they originated and showing varying number of
female founders for each of these populations. (See color figure.)

Among the Jews of Azerbajian, Georgia, Libya, Mumbai, India,
and Belmonte, Portugal, there are very few founder lineages
that account for the majority of mitochondrial haplotypes. A
single mother was sufficient to account for at least 40% of contemporary mitochondrial genomes. Among the Jews of Cochin
(south India) and Tunisia, two founding mothers account for
30% of the mitochondrial genomes. In a number of Jewish
communities, including the Bulgarian, Turkish, Moroccan, and
Ethiopian, there was no evidence for a narrow founder effect

or depletion of mitochondrial genomes from a genetic bottleneck. The Bulgarian, Turkish, and Moroccan communities all received large influxes of Jewish refugees following the Spanish Inquisition. The high degree of diversity observed today probably reflects the degree of diversity that was present among the Jews of Spain. The diversity observed among the Ethiopian Jews reflects the variety of maternal lineages that were present during the founding and propagation of this community in East Africa. By contrast, the Iranian, Iraqi, and Yemeni communities demonstrate a degree of diversity that is intermediate to that observed in the other groups. The communities were all founded at least 2,000 years ago. The mitochondrial genotypes reflect that the founding event was not a narrow one. In fact, there were at least six founding mothers in these populations. None of these populations is quite like the contemporary Ashkenazi Jews, who have a large contemporary population (8–9 million) but relatively few founders.

All of the populations, with the exception of the Indians and Ethiopians, had mitochondrial genomes that were of Middle Eastern origin. This demonstrates that Jewish origins have been determined not only by the flow of genes but also by the flow of ideas, although this does not exclude the flow of genes from some founder Jewish women in the formation of a new Jewish group. This observation provides some resolution to the queries of Fishberg and Jacobs for why Indian and Ethiopian Jews bear a physical resemblance to their local populations.

Few of the mitochondrial lineages are shared across population groups. This could support the observations of the famous twelfth-century Jewish traveler Benjamin of Tudela, who reported that the Jewish tribesmen in Persia and the Arabian Peninsula were the descendants of the Lost Tribes of Israel as each tribe could have had its own founding matriarchs. He wrote in his *Book of Travels*, "There are men of Israel in the land of Persia who say that in the mountains dwell four of the tribes of Israel, namely, the tribe of Dan, the tribe of Zevulun, the tribe of Asher, and the tribe of Naphtali."[145] About the Jews of Arabia, he wrote, "These tribesmen are of the tribes Reuven and Gad, and the half-tribe of Menasseh. Their seat of government is a great city surrounded by the mountains of the North." Benjamin's *Travels* were translated into many languages and inspired others to search for the independent kingdoms of the Ten Lost Tribes.

One mitochondrial lineage shared among Libyan and Tunisian Jews is X2e1a1a, which can be explained by the geographical proximity of these populations.[144] This lineage is also found among non-Jewish Tunisians, suggesting that it might have been transmitted from Jews to non-Jews in this country (or that some bearers may have converted to Islam). Sub-Saharan African lineages are quite rare among almost all Jewish groups, with the exception of Ethiopian and Yemenite Jews, perhaps reflecting the prevalence of these lineages among non-Jews in Ethiopia and Yemen. Some of these sub-Saharan African lineages, although rare among Jews, are nonetheless prevalent among North African Arabs and Berbers.

Among the Indian Jews, the common mitochondrial haplogroups resemble those that are commonly observed among other Indians. The Hg M5a2 that is found in many Cochin Jews is particularly frequent in the Indian state of Kerala, suggesting local origin.[144] The few H mitochondrial haplotypes that have been observed in the B'nei Israel of Mumbai have not been observed among non-Jewish Indians. Rather, they have been observed among Iranian and Iraqi Jews, suggesting limited female gene flow from those communities. The Cochin Jews also possess the mitochondrial U1 haplogroup that is present in several non-Ashkenazi Jewish communities but is otherwise not present in western India. These observations suggest that the two Indian Jewish communities still contain mitochondrial lineages that were brought by founders from the Middle East into India. Behar and coworkers have concluded that idea-flow, rather than gene flow, may have constituted the main basis for establishing Jewish communities in Ethiopia and India.

These results contrast with an earlier study in which geneticist Mark Thomas noted, "The results suggest that most Jewish communities were founded by relatively few women, that the founding process was independent in different geographic areas, and that subsequent genetic input from surrounding populations was limited on the female side."[146] What the more recent study shows is that the narrow founder effects that are observed for Ashkenazi Jews are not observed for the other numerically large Moroccan, Iranian, Iraqi, and Sephardic (Iberian Exile) communities. Rather, they are observed only for the smallest, most remote non-Ashkenazi Jewish communities, as one might expect. This disparity between Thomas and Behar reflects the evolution of genetic marker analysis with analysis of more markers, more populations, and larger population sample sizes, which leads to greater precision about the population's genetic histories. The observation of the remote communities of Georgia, Ajerbajian, and India sharing mitochondrial haplotypes with local populations substantiated Goldstein's scenario of Jewish men, perhaps traders along the Silk Road, establishing local communities and marrying local women.[123]

Thus, the genetic analysis of contemporary Jewish populations has provided indications about Jewish origins and relatedness of Jewish populations. For the most part, they tend to fit the expectations of Jewish history, origins in the Middle East, with Diaspora populations having specific founders. Despite high rates of historical endogamy within these populations, some admixture occurred across Jewish populations and with local populations. For some populations this was quite high, as Jacobs described in his entry about Ethiopian and B'nei Israel Jews in the *Jewish Encyclopedia*. The Jewish story is not unique, only longer.

The study of Jews is occurring against the backdrop of worldwide efforts to use Y-chromosomal and mitochondrial lineages as a basis for understanding the deep ancestry of all major human populations. Among the largest and most

significant of these efforts is the Geographic Project, a collaborative venture of the National Geographic Society, IBM,
and a team of scientists around the world.[147] They gather field
research data in collaboration with local indigenous and traditional peoples and enable the general public to join the project by purchasing Genographic Project Public participation
kits. Participation in the project is described as "anonymous,
non-medical, non-political, non-profit and non-commercial."
The results have been published in scientific journals, then
placed in the public domain.

The studies from the Genographic Project have followed
Y-chromosomal and mitochondrial genetic markers in exquisite detail, as they migrated and evolved during human history. Some of the results have been unanticipated, whereas
others have not. In a study entitled, "Y-chromosomal diversity in Lebanon is structured by recent historical events,"
a team from the Genographic Project could trace the Muslim
and Christian peopling of Lebanon.[121] They demonstrated
that male genetic variation within Lebanon was structured by
religious affiliation rather than by geography. Y-chromosome
haplogroup J other than J2 *(xJ2) was more frequent in
Lebanese Muslims than in Lebanese non-Muslims. As
noted previously, this Y-chromosomal type originated in the
Arabian Peninsula and its prevalence represents the Muslim
peopling of Lebanon in the sixth and seventh centuries.
The Western European haplogroup R1b was prevalent in
Lebanese Christians, representing the Crusader activity in the

eleventh to thirteenth centuries C.E. that introduced Western
European lineages into Lebanese Christians.

In another study entitled, "The dawn of human matrilineal diversity," a Genographic Project team demonstrated
a genealogical tree of maternal lineages composed of the
complete DNA sequence from the mitochondrial genomes
from 624 sub-Saharan Africans who all had the mitochondrial DNA L lineages.[148] Among the people that they studied were the Khoisan, a group of hunter-gatherers living in
South Africa who speak a click language thought to be ancestral to other languages. Their paternal and maternal lineages
are known to be among the most ancient. The results of
the Genographic Project team's study were quite striking
and shed new light into the time following Mitochondrial
Eve. The Khoisan matrilineal ancestry diverged from the rest
of the human mtDNA (*mt* signifies "mitochondrial") pool
about 90,000 to 150,000 years ago. At least five additional
maternal lineages existed during this period and have been
transmitted to people living in sub-Saharan Africa up to
the present. By the time of modern human dispersal out of
Africa approximately 60,000 to 70,000 years ago, a mini-
mum of 40 other evolutionarily successful lineages flourished in sub-Saharan Africa. Only at the beginning of the
Late Stone Age, about 40,000 years ago, were other lineages
brought into the pool of Khoisan mtDNA, so the Khoisan
lived in relative isolation for 100,000 years. This process
was accelerated in more recent times when people speaking

Bantu languages mixed with the Khoisan. This research suggests that early human populations in Africa lived in isolation and evolved separately.

The Genographic Project, along with others, has tapped into a consumer market for individuals who want to know their heritage. Often, it is for people who want to know whether individuals who share a surname are related to one another. In my family's case, we wanted to know whether all males with the Ostrer surname had a common paternal ancestor—they do not. It turns out to be us (my family) and them (the other Ostrers). Others may be looking for a male or female ancestor who was a Cohan, a king, or a Jew. A friend had asked me about availability of genetic testing to know her origins. She believed that her birth mother was a young, unmarried Jewish woman, based on her surname. She also believed that her adoption had been arranged by a physician who specialized in adoption of Jewish children by Jewish parents. Her adopted parents were observant and transmitted a love of Judaism. Although not a Bat Mitzvah in adolescence, she became one as an adult. She married two Jewish men, raised three Jewish children, including a child from overseas that she and her husband adopted. Her children attended a Jewish day school and she was an active congregant in a Reform synagogue. Not too long ago, she pointed out to me during a dinner at her house that she had not pursued mitochondrial DNA testing. I guessed that she was looking for encouragement from me, but her husband interjected, "If the results do not meet your expectations, you will probably be very disappointed. It is probably better for you not to be tested."

This genetic view of Jewish history may have seemed fanciful to Jacobs and to Eliot's readers, but in our era, it has captured our attention. Through the print media, public radio stories, and NOVA television series, we have become aware of the potential for genetic analysis to test and validate hypotheses about our own human history.

FOUR

TRIBES

If being Jewish were in the blood, then what better way to identify the markers of Jewishness than by studying blood itself? Blood-typing is more precise than anthropometry and specific blood groups are more prevalent than genetic diseases. Arthur Mourant, one of the foremost cataloguers of blood groups during the twentieth century was the champion of this approach (Figure 4.1). In his 1977 book, *The Genetics of the Jews*, Mourant explained the advantages to this approach:

> In popular anthropology since time immemorial, and in
> a more precise manner for more than a century, the vis-
> ible and physically measurable body characteristics preceded
> the hereditary blood characteristics as the principal human

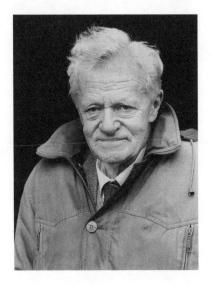

Figure 4.1. Photo of Arthur Mourant, English hematologist, and popularizer of the use of blood groups for performing population genetic studies, including among Jewish populations. Photograph copyright *Jersey Evening Post*. Used with permission.

taxonomic markers. Because of the precisely known mode of inheritance of blood characters, the latter have now super-seded them…The hereditary diseases are, in general, too rare to be of value in studies of limited population samples…[149]

Although Mourant was one of the great cataloguers of Jewish population genetics, his road to population genetics was long.[150] He started as an Oxford-trained geologist. As a member of the Geological Survey of Great Britain during the 1920s, he developed his skills as a cataloguer mapping the coal deposits in Lancashire. Unable to obtain an academic post in geology in

Depression-era Britain upon receiving his Ph.D. from Oxford
in 1931, he returned to his native island of Jersey and set up
a laboratory offering medical tests. Running that laboratory
was not satisfying, so in 1939, at age 34 years, he entered St.
Bartholomew's Medical College in London. Upon his gradua-
tion with a medical degree in 1943, he became a Medical Officer
in the National Blood Transfusion Service and rapidly became
a leader in the field. After the war, he became the Director of
the Medical Research Council's newly established Blood Group
Reference Laboratory, the international standard for the World
Health Organization.

A blood group (or blood type) is based on the presence
or absence of certain sugars, proteins, or fats on the sur-
faces of blood cells and other types of cells. The reason why
these exist has never been discerned, but differences in blood
groups limit the possibilities for blood transfusions—blood
can be transfused only for a compatible type. Transfusions
among individuals of noncompatible types result in transfusion reactions in which antibodies in the recipient's blood
break down the transfused red cells. The effects can be even
more dramatic in babies. Antibodies from the mother can
cross the placenta and cause the blood cells of the fetus to
break down. This might not be apparent during pregnancy,
because the placenta exerts a protective effect, filtering out
the toxic products derived from the broken-down blood cells.
After birth, this incompatibility of the baby's and mother's
blood groups might be manifest as *hemolytic disease of the newborn*,

in which the destroyed red blood cells release their oxygen-carrying pigment, hemoglobin. In turn, this is broken down into the yellow pigment bilirubin, causing severe jaundice in the baby. The correction for this condition is an exchange transfusion in which blood from a donor whose blood group is compatible with the *baby's* is used to completely replace the baby's blood volume. The replacement of the baby's red blood cells and the elimination of the antibodies from the mother correct this condition.

The presence of these antibodies was recognized first in 1901 by Karl Landsteiner, a Viennese pathologist. As he noted later in his Nobel Prize lecture of 1930:

> My experiment consisted of causing the blood serum and erythrocytes (red blood cells) of different human subjects to react with one another. The result was only to some extent as expected. With many samples there was no perceptible alteration, in other words the result was exactly the same as if the blood cells had been mixed with their own serum, but frequently a phenomenon known as agglutination—in which the serum causes the cells of the alien individual to group into clusters—occurred.[151]

Following Landsteiner's lead, serum banks were created that used collected serum from individuals of known blood groups and used these sera to test new individuals to determine their types. It was to a laboratory with just such a serum bank that Mourant headed after World War II.

In the ABO system, there are four blood groups: A, B, AB, and O—O represents the absence of A or B. People with the O group are also known as "universal donors," because they can give blood to anyone. ABO and other blood groups are genetically encoded. The ABO system actually comprises three forms of the same gene, A, B, and O. O people receive the O form from both parents. People with the A group might have inherited A from both parents or A from one parent and O from the other. People with the B group might have inherited B from both parents or B from one parent and O from the other. People with AB inherited A from one parent and B from the other.

The study of ABO blood groups made it immediately clear that there are different frequencies among different peoples.[152] In Europe, the average frequency is 40% O, 40% A, 15% B, and 5% AB. In other populations, the balance changes. Among Native Americans, virtually all are type O, with the exception of some Canadian tribes that have a high incidence of A. B is simply not observed. Blood groups represent genetic markers that have provided a basis for studying the origins and relatedness of human populations.[131]

Mourant was among the first to appreciate the utility of using blood groups as population genetic markers and became one of the great cataloguers of blood groups among the world's populations. As he noted, cataloguing blood groups provided a distinctive basis for examining human differences that were not based on physical traits (head shape, height, skin and eye color) that were fairly imprecise or on genetic diseases that individually were relatively rare. In addition to ABO, RH was a useful blood group for cataloging populations, because the highest frequency of RH-negative is found among European populations, averaging 10% to 15%. Among the Basques of Spain and France, it is even higher.[153] The Basque hematologist Michel Angelo Etcheverry suggested that the Basques of today might be the descendants of founders whose frequency of RH-negative was as high as 100%.[154]

The history of the discovery of the RH blood group is almost as remarkable as that of ABO. Landsteiner and Weiner identified the RH blood group in 1937, some 40 years after Landsteiner's original demonstration of the ABO group.[155] They observed that human serum could produce a clumping reaction of the red blood cells of the rhesus monkey, but the clumping reaction was produced by those people who did not have this *Rhesus* blood group, the RH-negative individuals. Serum from those who had the RH blood group did not produce the clumping reaction.[155] In 1940, 3 years after the identification of the RH blood group, New York pediatrician Philip Levine observed that incompatibility of the RH blood group was a frequent cause of the disorder *erythroblastosis fetalis* (large fetal red cells)—also a cause of hemolytic disease of the newborn.[156] Levine observed that RH-positive blood cells from the fetus can cross the placenta at birth. As a result, the mother becomes sensitized to the fetal blood cells and produces antibodies. In a subsequent pregnancy, the mother's antibodies cross the placenta and destroy the red blood cells of the RH-positive fetus, producing severe anemia, an outcrop of large red cells, and heart failure and edema. The RH blood group is also genetically transmitted, with RH-negative representing a recessive trait. RH-negative mothers and fathers cannot have RH-positive fetuses. Landsteiner appreciated the genetic transmission and that fetal sensitization might disclose nonpaternity.[151] The biological father's blood group might be RH-positive, whereas the husband's blood group might be RH-negative. The RH-negative husband would be suspicious that an RH-positive fetus with *erythroblastosis fetalis* was not his child.[157] Since Landsteiner's time, a treatment has been developed for *erythroblastosis fetalis*. It can now be prevented by treating RH-negative mothers with *Rhogam*, an antibody against the RH blood group that will destroy the RH-positive red blood cells in the mother's circulation, reducing risks for both fetuses and mothers.[158]

Mourant used this information to develop a blood group catalog of different Jewish groups.[149] Based on his lifelong interest in the history of the Jews and the Jewish Diasporas, Mourant was very motivated to develop such a catalog. He attributed this interest to his first school teacher, a British Israelite who believed that all the British people were descended from the Lost Tribes of Israel. As the English anthropologist Tudor Parfitt has noted, "In England, as in other parts of Britain, however, there was a long-running discourse celebrating the notion that the English themselves were literally of Jewish extraction and that the ancestors of the English people were in fact Israelites."[159] He went on to note, "British Israelism became a sanctification and validation of the British Empire."[159] Mourant's interest in studying the Jewish populations of Israel was invigorated by Sheba's 1961 conference in Jerusalem. In the proceedings of the conference, he noted, "There is here a unique opportunity for studying human evolution in action."[39] Over the next decade, he put this into practice and produced his detailed catalog, *The Genetics of the Jews.*[149]

Mourant's catalog had varying data for the different blood groups and for other genetic marker systems (including G6PD). He recognized that the ABO and RH blood groups were the most important for causing transfusion reactions and for identifying differences in populations. He also catalogued other known blood groups, including the M and N groups that he had been the first to identify. He concluded that the blood group data correlated with the known facts of Jewish history—although population geneticists at the time and today would agree that it is hard to draw major conclusions from a single genetic marker system. The major Jewish communities were relatively homogeneous, yet distinct from one another. Each of the communities bore some resemblance to the indigenous people who resided within the Jewish Diaspora community. In Mourant's words, "Each major Jewish community as a whole bears some resemblance to indigenous peoples of the region where it first developed."[39] The Iraqi Jews who had an historic claim to being the descendants of the Jews of the Babylonian captivity did

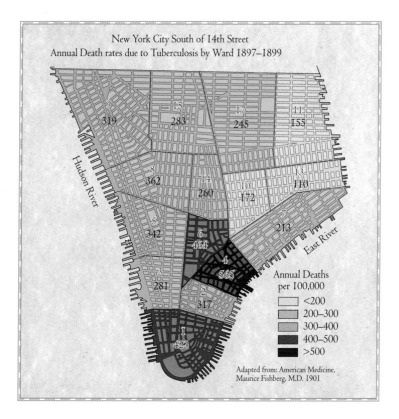

New York City South of 14th Street
Annual Death rates due to Tuberculosis by Ward 1897–1899

Hudson River

East River

9
319

15
283

17
245

11
155

8
362

14
260

10
172

13
110

5
342

6
464

7
213

3
281

4
565

2
317

1
423

Annual Deaths
per 100,000

<200
200–300
300–400
400–500
>500

Adapted from: American Medicine,
Maurice Fishberg, M.D. 1901

Figure 1.2. Fishberg's map of annual tuberculosis death rates by ward in
New York City south of 14th Street 1897 1899. Note that the rates
were lowest in the wards that had the highest proportion of
Jews—the 10th, 11th, and 13th.

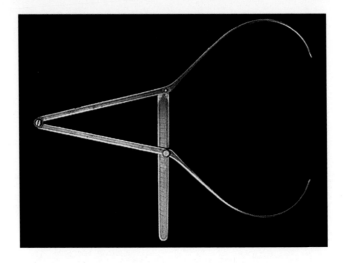

Figure 1.3. Calipers similar to those used by Maurice Fishberg and other physical anthropologists for measuring head proportions to determine cephalic indices.

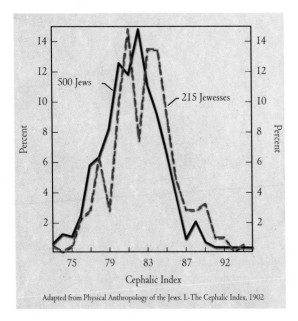

Adapted from Physical Anthropology of the Jews. I.-The Cephalic Index, 1902

Figure 1.4. Fishberg's graphs for the cephalic indices of Jewish men and women. A cephalic index of 81–83 is indicative of brachycephaly or round-headedness. Note that the Jewish men had a curve with a single peak and fairly narrow width, suggesting a homogeneous distribution. The cephalic index distribution for Jewish women almost completely overlapped that of men but had two peaks, suggesting two possible groups.

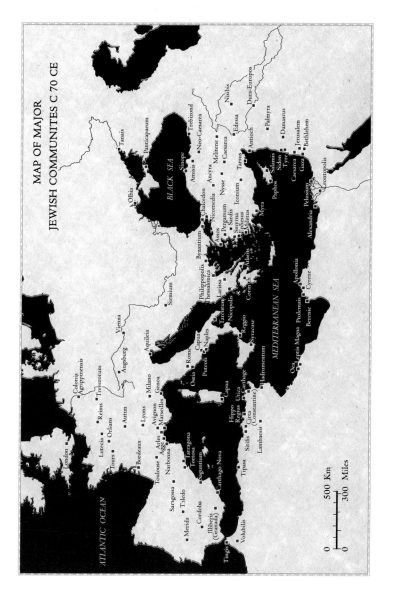
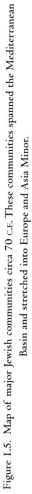

MAP OF MAJOR
JEWISH COMMUNITES C 70 CE

ATLANTIC OCEAN

London
Colonia
Agrippinensis
Lutecia ■ Reims ■ Treverorum
Tours ■ Orléans
Bordeaux Autun
Lyons
Toulouse ■ Avignon ■ Milano
Arles ■ Marseilles ■ Genoa
Narbonna Agge

Augsburg
Vienna

Aquileia

Sirmium

Tanais

Olbia
Panticapaeum

BLACK SEA

Sinope
Amisa ■ Neo-Caesarea
Ancyra ■ Melitene
Nicomedia ■ Nysse ■ Caesarea
Sardis ■ Iconium
Smyrna ■ Ephesus
Assos Pergamum
Byzantium
Chalcedon

Trebizond

Nisibis
Edessa ■ Dura-Europos
Palmyra
Antioch ■ Damascus
Tarsus
Salamis ■ Sidon
Paphos ■ Tyre
Caesarea ■ Jerusalem
Gaza ■ Bethlehem
Pelusium
Leontopolis

Saragossa
Toledo
Illiberis
(Granada)
Volubilis
Cordoba
Merida
Tingis

Tarragona
Fortosa
Saguntum
Carthago Nova
Tipasa
Sitifis
Lambaesis

Hippo
Regius ■ Utica
Cirta ■ Carthage
(Constantine)

Hadrumetum

Oea
Aegis Magna
Berenic ■ Ptolemais
Apollonia
Cyrene

Rome
Ostia ■ Capua
Puteoli ■ Naples
Capua
Reggio
Syracuse

Tarentum
Nicopolis
Larissa
Thessalonica
Philippopolis

Corinth
Athens

Myra
Miletus

MEDITERRANEAN SEA

0 ┣━━━┫ 500 Km
0 ┣━━━┫ 300 Miles

Figure I.5. Map of major Jewish communities circa 70 C.E. These communities spanned the Mediterranean
Basin and stretched into Europe and Asia Minor.

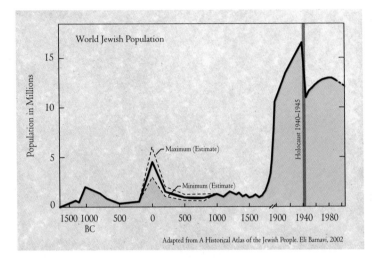

Figure I.6. Changes in Jewish population size over time. The Jewish
population numbered 6 million in Classical Antiquity, a number
that was not matched again until the 1800s.

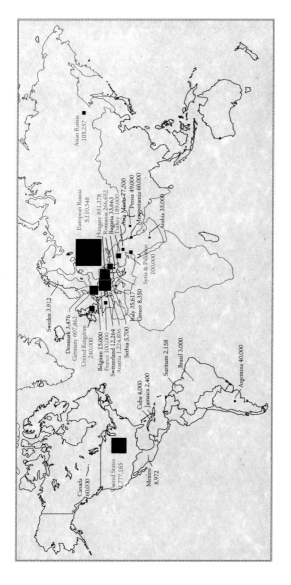

Figure I.7. Map of major Jewish communities circa 1900 C.E. The sizes of the squares correspond to the sizes of the Jewish populations. Virtually all Diaspora communities were still inhabited by Jews. Almost 2 million Jews lived in the United States by that time.

Pattern of Transmission of an X-linked Disorder

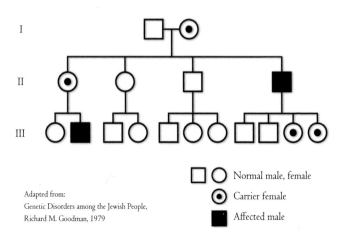

Adapted from:
Genetic Disorders among the Jewish People,
Richard M. Goodman, 1979

□ ○ Normal male, female
◉ Carrier female
■ Affected male

**Figure 2.3. Pedigree of X-linked inheritance for G6PD deficiency.
Note the absence of transmission from fathers to sons.**

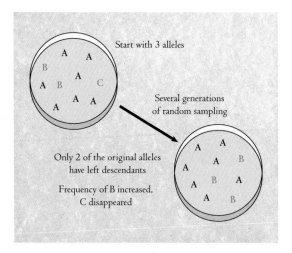

**Figure 2.5. Genetic drift in small populations results in random
fluctuations and increase or decrease in mutant allele
frequency from one generation to the next.**

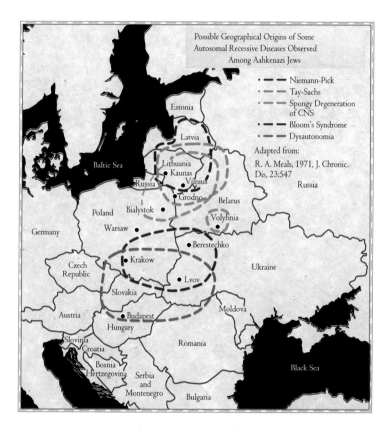

Figure 2.6. Richard Goodman's map of founder effects for common Ashkenazi Jewish disease mutations, based on reported places of residence of grandparents of grandparents of affected children.

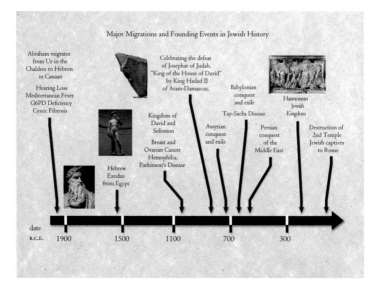

Figure 2.7. Early timeline showing coalescence of founder mutations and comparing these with events in Jewish history.

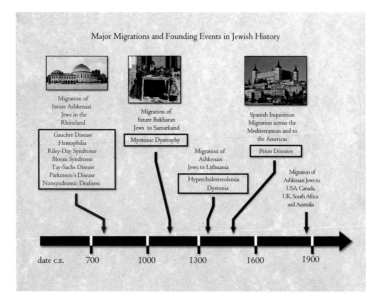

Figure 2.8. Later timeline showing coalescence of founder mutations and comparing these with events in Jewish history.

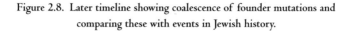

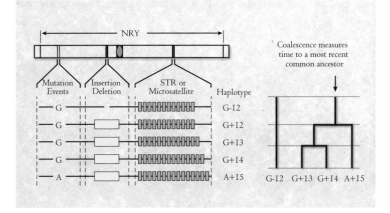

Figure 3.2. The combination of markers genotyped at polymorphic sites anywhere on the Y-chromosome of each male is referred to as a haplotype. Coalescence of the various markers measures the time to a most recent common ancestor.

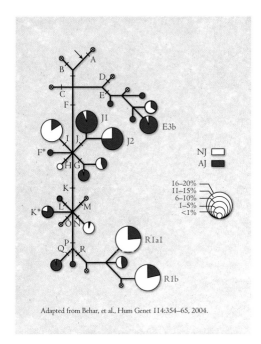

Adapted from Behar, et al., Hum Genet 114:354–65, 2004.

Figure 3.3. Y-chromosomal haplogroups among Ashkenazi Jews demonstrate descent from a discrete set of founders.

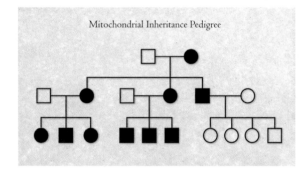

Figure 3.4. Pedigree of mitochondrial inheritance demonstrating maternal transmission to offspring.

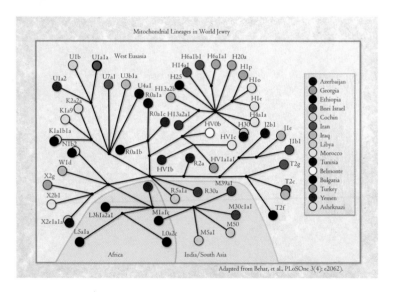

Figure 3.5. Mitochondrial lineages among World Jewry and geographical locales from which they originated and showing varying number of female founders for each of these populations.

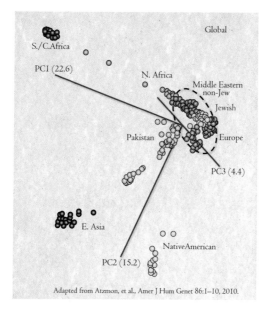

Adapted from Atzmon, et al., Amer J Hum Genet 86:1–10, 2010.

Figure 4.3. Principle component (PC) analysis of world populations showing major population groups from Africa, Eurasia, America, East Asia, and Oceania. PC1 distinguishes Sub-Saharan ancestry; PC2 distinguishes East Asian ancestry and PC3 distinguishes European, Middle Eastern, and North African ancestry. The Mizrahi (Middle Eastern) and European Jewish populations form a cluster between the Middle Eastern and European non-Jewish populations.

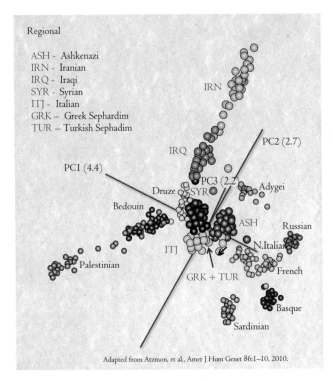

Regional

ASH - Ashkenazi
IRN - Iranian
IRQ - Iraqi
SYR - Syrian
ITJ - Italian
GRK — Greek Sephardim
TUR — Turkish Sephadim

Adapted from Atzmon, et al., Amer J Hum Genet 86:1–10, 2010.

Figure 4.4. Principle component analysis demonstrating that Ashkenazi, Sephardic, and Mizrahi Jews form a distinctive population cluster that is closely related to Middle Eastern non-Jewish and European populations. Within this larger cluster, each of the Jewish populations forms its own subcluster.

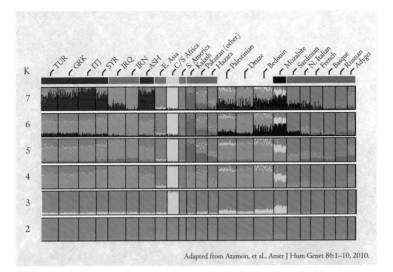

Adapted from Atzmon, et al., Amer J Hum Genet 86:1–10, 2010.

Figure 4.5. Population structure analysis of imputed ancestries based on analysis of hundreds of thousands of genetic markers and demonstrating a high degree of European admixture among Ashkenazi, Sephardic, Italian, and Syrian Jews.

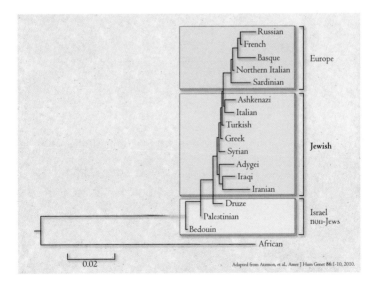

Adapted from Atzmon, et al., Amer J Hum Genet 86:1–10, 2010.

Figure 4.6. Neighbor joining tree demonstrating genetic sharing among Jewish groups and a split between European/Syrian Jews and Middle Eastern Iraqi and Iranian Jews that was timed to have occurred approximately 2500 years ago.

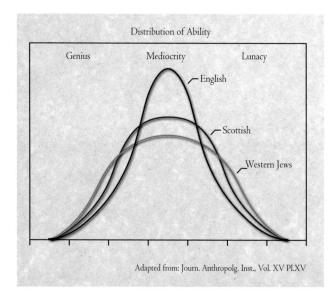

Figure 5.2. Joseph Jacobs' observations about IQ distributions in different populations, allegedly demonstrating a higher proportion of "genius" and "lunacy" among Scots and Jews.

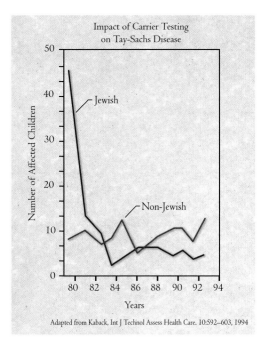

Impact of Carrier Testing
on Tay-Sachs Disease

Number of Affected Children

Jewish

Non-Jewish

Years

Adapted from Kaback, Int J Technol Assess Health Care. 10:592–603, 1994

Figure 5.3. Effect of genetic carrier screening on reducing the incidence of
Tay-Sachs disease. With screening, Tay-Sachs went from being a
Jewish-predominant to a non-Jewish-predominant disease.

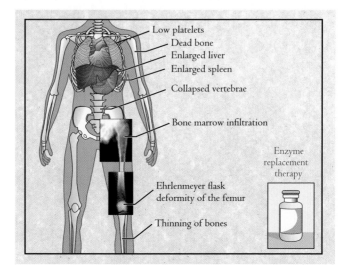

Figure 5.4. Effects of treating Gaucher disease with enzyme-replacement
therapy with alleviation of many of the pathological features.

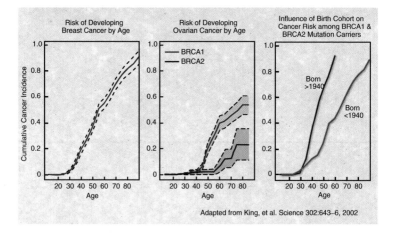

Adapted from King, et al. Science 302:643–6, 2002

Figure 5.5. Significant discoveries from studying *BRCA1/2* mutations in
Ashkenazi Jewish populations—(Left) similar risk of developing breast cancer by
age 80 years, regardless of whether a woman is a *BRCA1* or *BRCA2* mutation
carrier; (Center) Higher risk of developing ovarian cancer by age 80 years,
if a woman is a *BRCA1* rather than *BRCA2* mutation carrier; (Right)
Apparent earlier onset of breast cancer if a woman was born after 1940.

not deviate markedly from the surrounding non-Jewish people. The Yemenite Jews were distinct from other Middle Eastern Jews but had a close resemblance to the Arabs of the Arabian Peninsula. The Ashkenazi Jews were distinct from the Turkic peoples of Central Asia, people who are thought to be related to and possibly descended from the Khazars. This tended to negate Koestler's concept of a Khazarian origin for Ashkenazi, a concept he popularized in his book, *The Thirteenth Tribe*.[36]

A drawback to the study of blood groups was that, individually, they were not very informative about peoples' ancestry—Mourant recognized that his data were insufficient to infer the blood groups of the original Jews of Palestine. He did not have methods for combining data from several different blood group systems to draw statistical conclusions; thus, most of his conclusions were drawn on observations from the ABO system. This shortcoming was remedied by the development of mathematical methods that combined data from several different blood groups or other genetic markers that demonstrated variation in human populations. The combination of markers was more informative about ancestry than each marker individually.

The leader of this effort to develop combinatorial methods was Luigi Luca Cavalli-Sforza, an Italian nobleman and physician. Cavalli-Sforza went on to become one of the leading population geneticists of the twentieth century, not only for his development of methods that were adopted by other population geneticists but also for his books and speeches that popularized the study of human origins and evolution. He noted,

"I was attracted to the study of evolution by a consideration that I think of as aesthetic: the sheer beauty of the theory of evolution."[160] Cavalli-Sforza trained in medicine in Italy during World War II and then in genetics at Cambridge University. Between 1948 and 1950, he worked with Sir Ronald Fisher, the father of modern statistics and one of the outstanding geneticists of the twentieth century. Fisher was one of the creators of the modern synthesis, the theory that provided a genetic basis for evolution by natural selection.[161] Fisher's emphasis on studying blood groups as a basis for characterizing genetic differences between human populations influenced the direction that Cavalli-Sforza selected for his own work.

Cavalli-Sforza supposed that if enough data were gathered on many different blood group (and other) genes, that it might be possible to reconstruct the entire genetic history of humans. This accumulation of large quantities of data would provide a clearer understanding than that obtained sometimes intuitively using a single gene. Cavalli-Sforza developed analytical methods that would quantify the differences between populations. He was convinced that the field would progress rapidly, because of the large number of researchers working on blood groups and other genetic variations that were being discovered at that time.

In 1960, Cavalli-Sforza invited Anthony Edwards, his fellow trainee in Ronald Fisher's laboratory at Cambridge, to work with him in Pavia, Italy. Edwards was an expert not only on population genetics and statistics but also on data processing. The timing of this association was fortuitous, because the University of Pavia had a new Olivetti computer that was available for their almost exclusive use. Working together, they developed two methods for analyzing combined genetic datasets—genetic distances and dendritic trees. Genetic distances represented the data of gene frequencies in a population as a line or vector in space.[162–163] Two populations that had similar origins and, thus, similar data for their set of genetic markers have lines of similar length and direction. Therefore, the distance between them is short. Two populations that had widely disparate origins have very different frequencies for their sets of markers, and these were represented as lines of unequal length and different directions. The distance between them was long. Populations with the greatest distances were the most disparate, just as one would expect. Using RH as an example, if the gene frequencies for RH-negative were 20% among Basques, 15% among English, and 2% among Chinese, then a simple genetic distance could be 5% between Basques and English, 18% between Basques and Chinese, and 13% between English and Chinese. In fact, their formula was more complex, incorporating data for many genes. Using this method, all populations could be represented together graphically, facilitating comparisons.

The other method that Cavalli-Sforza and Edwards developed was dendritic trees—trees with branches.[162] The most closely related populations were on the same twig; the most closely related groups were on the same branch. The distance between the branching points was a measure of the time when one population broke off from another. Cavalli-Sforza and

Edwards discovered that many different genetic trees were possible, so they developed the statistical method of parsimony. The parsimonious tree was the one that required the fewest branches to explain the observed genetic data. Thus, Cavalli-Sforza's methods provided a way for analyzing the compendium of data that Mourant collected.

Cavalli-Sforza has summarized his work in this way:

> During 1961 and 1962, we brought together data published on about fifteen populations, three per continent, dealing with a total of twenty genetic variations. All the data were on blood groups: ABO, RH and three other systems...We assessed the genetic distances between pairs of populations on the basis of these data, for each of the 105 combinations offered by two-by-two comparisons. This gave us the most rational tree possible using the available data and applying our specially developed reconstruction methods. Our first attempt is still relatively correct today, despite the relatively small number of genes used. Populations from the same continent tended to fall close together, and this was a good sign, because it was reasonable to expect that populations from the same continent should form close knit clusters.[160]

The Native Americans tended to be related to the Eskimos and more distantly to the Koreans. Cavalli-Sforza took this as a favorable sign, because both Native Americans and Eskimos are Mongolian in origin and arrived in America from Eastern Asia via Siberia and Alaska. The Europeans were an intermediate group between Africans and Asians. The people at the extremes of human variation were the Africans and the New Guineans and Australian Aborigines. Plotting the tree on a world map provided an indication of the routes taken by modern humans during their geographic expansion. Cavalli-Sfoza and his coworkers assumed that the forks in their tree corresponded to the separation between two peoples in historical terms, to the time when one group moved far enough away from another to restrict contact severely. The sequences of the branches corresponded to the actual splits, and the position and length of the branches corresponded to the time when the splits occurred.

Subsequently, the statistical methods that Cavalli-Sforza pioneered for analyzing blood groups and other genetic markers were employed for studying Jewish populations. In his own study of Jewish and non-Jewish populations that he performed with Dorit Carmelli, Cavalli-Sforza analyzed 12 Jewish populations and 20 non-Jewish populations using the ABO, RH, MN blood groups and the variable haptoglobin genetic marker, haptoglobin being a protein that carries hemoglobin in blood.[164] Their study, in turn, was followed by many others. Virtually all of the studies agreed that most Jewish populations had a Middle Eastern origin. Where they differed was in the degree of admixture that they identified with local populations. A study by Morton and his coworkers drew the conclusion of substantial admixture between Jewish and neighboring non-Jewish populations,[165] whereas studies by Bonne-Tamir, Karlin, Livshits, Kobyliansky, and Wijsman determined that there was much less.[166-170] These studies demonstrated a greater genetic similarity between most pairs of Jewish populations than between paired Jewish and neighboring non-Jewish communities. Unfortunately, these studies were not entirely comparable. They differed in the number and provenance of the Jewish and non-Jewish populations and in the number and identity of the genetic markers analyzed. At the time, Bonne-Tamir wrote, "The difficulties of assessing relationships on the basis of a few selected differences and the need for careful interpretation of similarities are emphasized."[171] In the 1990s, Bonne-Tamir facilitated these comparisons by creating the National Laboratory for the Genetics of Israeli Populations, a national repository for human cell lines that represented the ethnic variation of the Israeli populations—Jewish, Arab, and Druze (Figure 4.2).

During the heyday of blood group and other genetic marker studies, anthropologist Rafael Patai and his geneticist daughter Jennifer Patai-Wing decided that they had sufficient evidence to refute the earlier arguments of Jacobs and other physical anthropologists that the Jews constituted a race of people. In fact, they called their book *The Myth of the Jewish Race.*[172] Rather than arguing on the basis of head shape, height, and skin color, as Fishberg and Boas had done, they used the emerging data about blood groups and other genetic markers. Confining themselves to Mourant's data, they observed that the ABO data revealed great diversity among different groups of Jews. Among the Jews in Asia, the ABO gene frequencies were very heterogeneous.

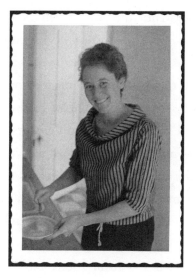

Figure 4.2. Photo of Batsheva Bonne-Tamir, Israeli geneticist,
who performed population genetic studies aimed at identifying the origins and
relatedness of Jewish groups. Bonne-Tamir established the National Laboratory
for the Genetics of Israeli Populations, a biorepository that made a
number of subsequent population genetic studies possible.

In fact, for the Patais, the differences were so great that they deemed that the Jews were not a homogeneous group—or a race. Yet, the Patais did not take advantage of the methods that were developed by Cavalli-Sforza and Edwards to analyze multiple genetic markers simultaneously. New insights were developed only in recent years through the analysis of entire genomes, fragments of which might be shared within a particular Diaspora Jewish group, among Jewish groups, or among Jews and non-Jews. Such analyses became possible during the latter part of the twentieth century, when the science of human genomics, the study of entire genomes, was created.

Genomics was created through the efforts of the Human Genome Project, the Big Science project of recent times.[173–174] As a result of this project, the content of the human genome was mapped and sequenced, and differences throughout the entire genome—not just Y chromosomal and mitochondrial—were identified. Among the differences that were identified were copy number variants (CNVs) and single nucleotide polymorphisms (SNPs), variations in the number of copies of a gene or a DNA sequence along a chromosome.[175–176] CNVs were found to vary in size from 960 to more than 3.4 million base pairs. Both SNPs and CNVs account for much of the common variation in human genomes, with SNPs accounting for 83% and CNVs for 17%. Other sources of variation also exist. Among these are rare variants that occur in less than 1% of the members of a population and short tandem repeats, a set of markers that gained popularity in the 1990s because they were easy for geneticists to identify and test on a large scale.[177]

Short-tandem repeat have the property of being comprised of runs of repeated bases of DNA—dinucleotide (such as CA), trinucleotides (such as CAG), and tetranucleotides (such as CAGA). Thus, on one region of a chromosome, an individual might have 10 copies of CA, 20 copies of CAG, and 30 copies of CAGA, whereas on his other, corresponding chromosome in the pair, he might have 12 copies of CA, 22 copies of

CAG, and 32 copies of CAGA. Thousands of these markers are scattered throughout the genome, and much of the success with identifying disease-predisposing genes in the 1990s mapped the gene between clusters of these markers. The markers also had the property of being informative about ancestry—different sizes of repeats for a given marker tended to be found in different populations. For a given CA repeat, it might tend to be short in Africans, longer in Europeans, and longer still in Asians.

The companion to the identification of these markers was the development of new methods for studying populations. Among these was *Structure*, a method developed by the geneticist Jonathan Pritchard while he was completing his training at Oxford University.[178] *Structure* analyzes a set of genetic data and determine how well they might be explained by having one, two, or more ancestral populations to the groups under analysis. It can also determine whether any given individual is likely to have descended from one or more of these groups and what fraction of his or her ancestry has been contributed by these ancestral groups.

Working with Noah Rosenberg, Marcus Feldman, and several other geneticists, Pritchard used a set of 377 short-tandem repeat markers to study 1,056 people from 52 populations with a worldwide distribution.[179] The results were both expected and startling. They observed that these populations clustered into six groups. Five of these clusters corresponded to geographic regions from which these populations came—Africa, Eurasia, America, East Asia, and Oceania (Pacific Islands; Figure 4.3). These clusters represented what might have been called races in

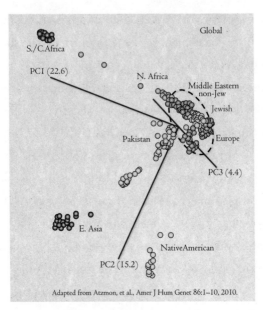

Adapted from Atzmon, et al., Amer J Hum Genet 86:1–10, 2010.

Figure 4.3. Principle component (PC) analysis of world populations showing major population groups from Africa, Eurasia, America, East Asia, and Oceania. PCI distinguishes Sub-Saharan ancestry; PC2 distinguishes East Asian ancestry and PC3 distinguishes European, Middle Eastern, and North African ancestry. The Mizrahi (Middle Eastern) and European Jewish populations form a cluster between the Middle Eastern and European non-Jewish populations. (See color figure.)

the past, or the "continental groups" that population geneticists Jorde, Tishkoff, and Risch had written about more recently. The sixth group was comprised of the Kalash, a people who speak an Indo-European language and live in the Northwest Frontier Province of Pakistan, apparently in relative isolation. This unexpected finding anticipated the possibility of identifying another genetic isolate in their next study.

Rosenberg, Pritchard, Feldman, and a different group of collaborators then applied their methods to the study of six Jewish groups (Ashkenazi, Ethiopian, Iraqi, Libyan, Moroccan, and Yemenite) and two non-Jewish Middle Eastern groups (Druze and Palestinian Arabs).[180] By comparison with their previous study, this one was relatively modest. Based on previous knowledge of Jewish population genetics, one might have expected the Yemenite or Ethiopian Jews to stand out from the other groups. Both claimed to have been descended from King Solomon and the Queen of Sheba. Both claimed to have been descended from the Ten Lost Tribes taken into captivity by the Assyrians, then dispersed. In fact, that was not what they observed at all. As they noted, "We found that the Libyan Jewish group retains genetic signatures distinguishable from those of the other populations, in agreement with some historical records on the relative isolation of this community. The Libyan Jewish appellation labeled not only a cultural group, but also a genetic isolate." In fact, Bonne-Tamir made a similar observation some 20 years earlier by studying blood groups. She observed:

> Blood groups, serum proteins, and red-cell enzyme frequencies were determined on a random sample of 148 Libyan Jews now settled in Israel. Comparisons with data on Libyan non-Jews show significant differences in most systems, implying maintenance of a high degree of genetic isolation of the Jewish group from surrounding populations.

The relative lack of the African component in their gene pool shows that they have interbred very little, if at all, with their [Sub-Saharan African] neighbours.[181]

The history of the Libyan Jews supports Bonne-Tamir's contention. This population was formed a long time ago (326 BCE) and grew to be quite large during Roman times.[93] During the first century of the Common Era, the Jewish historian Josephus recorded the presence of 500,000 Jews in the Libyan city of Cyrenaica. The population then went through a series of bottlenecks starting with the revolts against the Roman rulers from 115 to 118 CE, whereby its size diminished then increased. The Libyan Jews may have admixed with Berber tribes, among whom they established a process of Judaization. Over the past 400 years, the Libyan Jews were mostly isolated from all other Jewish populations. Jews left Libya and migrated to Israel following the Israeli War of Independence and the creation of the Jewish state in 1948—indeed, nearly 27,000 Libyan Jews settled in Israel.[182]

Once in Israel, some unusual genetic diseases not found in other Jewish groups were identified. Among the most unusual was the heritable form of Mad Cow (or Creutzfeld-Jacob) Disease.[183] As described earlier, The affected Libyan Jews were found to have a mutation in the prion gene, the gene that encodes the protein particle that can cause the transmissible form of Mad Cow Disease.[184]

In recent years, the genome-wide analyses that Pritchard, Rosenberg, and Feldman undertook with microsatellite markers have been surpassed by studies comparing entire genomes using several hundred-thousand genetic markers. These studies were facilitated by the the Human Genome Project's offshoot, the International HapMap Consortium, which defined the common SNPs and CNVs in representative Europeans, East Asians, and West Africans.[185] The SNP analysis demonstrated the block-like structure ("haplotype") in which these variants are inherited (the "HapMap"). This study showed that a typical haplotype is comprised of 5,000 to 20,000 bases of DNA. It is flanked on either side by "hotspots of recombination," sites that tend to be reshuffled when an egg cell or a sperm cell is formed. The presence of these hotspots preserves a structure that would be lost if the recombination occurred at random.

Several insights from the International HapMap Consortium described the general nature of human population genetics. Most of the common variants identified arose historically from single mutational events; therefore, these are associated with variants nearby that were present on the ancestral chromosome on which it occurred. Only a few of the possible haplotypes at each region of the genome have been observed, indicating limited diversity among all people. Nonetheless, the variation is great enough so that the sharing of SNPs, CNVs, and haplotypes defines the genetic history of a population. By using the large numbers of markers generated by the International HapMap Consortium, the amount of diversity within that population can be measured and the relatedness of one population to another can be determined with a greater degree of precision than Cavalli-Sforza,

Pritchard, or others could have achieved previously. Markers found at higher frequencies in certain populations are informative of ancestry for that population. Within the populations studied, 10% to 30% of pairs of individuals share at least one region of extended genetic identity arising from recent shared ancestry. This is genetic representation of the degree of relatedness between any two people in a population, although the actual degree of relatedness can be estimated more precisely by the number of shared segments.[186]

Recently, Cavalli-Sforza and his associates analyzed 938 unrelated individuals from 51 populations of the Human Genome Diversity Panel with 650,000 SNPs and discerned six ancestral populations: African, Middle Eastern, South/Central Asian, East Asian, Oceanian, and American.[176] With these additional markers, the Kalash were no longer observed as a separate population, and Middle Eastern ancestry was now discernable in some populations. Although Jews were not studied, the Bedouins, Palestinians, and Druze were all shown to have Middle Eastern as well as European and Central/South Asian ancestry—the proportions varying in each population. The genetic markers were most likely to be heterozygous among people from sub-Saharan Africa, less so in other populations. Overall the findings were compatible with the well-known model of humans originating and having the opportunity to accumulate the greatest genetic variation in southern Africa. Subsequently, they migrated north and out of Africa to found progenitor populations in new geographical locales, with many founding events discernable in the genomes of these populations.

A similar approach was used by Carlos Bustamante and his associates to study the populations of Europe.[187] Despite the considerable genetic similarity of European populations, Bustamante and associates observed a close correspondence between genetic and geographic distances of these populations. In fact, when the European populations were plotted on the basis of distance in two dimensions, they could be readily overlaid onto the map of Europe with Scandinavians in the North, English, Scottish, and Irish in the Northwest; Spanish and Portuguese in the Southwest; Italians in the South; Greeks and Turks in the Southeast; Russians and Poles in the East; and German and Swiss in the Center. The authors noted, "An individual's DNA can be used to infer their geographic origin with surprising accuracy—often to within a few hundred kilometers."

Understanding genetic ancestry is critical to contemporary genetic studies that associate genetic variants with human traits. Mistaking the ancestry of individuals in genetic studies can lead to errors in determining whether a particular gene has had a role in causing a trait or disease among the participants of the study. When performing such a study, the cases with the trait and the controls without should have the same ancestry. Having cases with Swedish ancestry and controls with Italian ancestry represents precisely this kind of mismatch. A study in which a difference is observed for the frequency of the marker in cases and controls may be interpreted as the marker's having a causal role for the trait, when actually it is demonstrating the difference in ancestry between the two groups. Through the use of genome-wide data or from a smaller set of ancestry-informative markers, the individuals who do not match can be excluded from the study. Alternatively, mathematical methods can be used to revise the frequency data so that they would represent the situation in which all participants had the same ancestry. It was just such a quest to define the differences in ancestry that led to three studies comparing Ashkenazi Jews with other people of European heritage.

These studies confirmed that the differences in European ancestry observed by Bustamante and associates in European populations were equally applicable to Americans whose ancestors came from different parts of Europe. Alkes Price, Michael Seldin, and their associates discerned that the major variation among European-Americans occurred along the northwest–southeast geographic line of European ancestry, with Ashkenazi Jews tending to cluster with people of southeastern European ancestry.[188–189] Yet, additional analysis readily distinguished people with Ashkenazi Jewish ancestry from those with southeastern European ancestry. Both Price and Seldin identified sets of genetic markers that could reliably discern ancestry and be used to correct for differences if Scandinavian-Americans, Italian-Americans, or Ashkenazi Jewish Americans were overrepresented in the cases or controls, and thus, there was not matching of ancestry between these two groups. Goldstein and his collaborators carried these observations a step further by showing that a set of ancestry-informative markers could perfectly distinguish Ashkenazi Jewish Americans from European-Americans. They wrote, "We show that, at least in the context of the studied sample, it is possible to predict full Ashkenazi Jewish ancestry with 100 percent sensitivity and 100 percent specificity..."[190] These observations are reminiscent of Fishberg's statement that it is possible to pick out one Jew from among 1,000 individuals without difficulty. Goldstein's study was unable to identify people with 1, 2, or 3 Jewish grandparents with the same degree of certainty as those with four Jewish grandparents, although other methods of analysis might.

My goal as a geneticist has not been to develop metrics for who will enjoy the benefits of membership in the club but, rather, to understand the history of Jews from their genomes and to understand the genetic basis for diseases among Jewish people. The recruitment and collection started more than a decade ago, first in New York and then in Rome. I had gone to Rome to undertake a study of a non-Jewish neurogenetic condition, hereditary sensory and autonomic neuropathy (HSAN) type IV. This condition shares some similarity with familial dysautonomia (FD) or HSAN type III, a neurogenetic condition found almost exclusively among Ashkenazi Jews. My NYU colleague, Felicia Axelrod, had been the leading caregiver and investigator of children with FD for the previous three decades. She had expanded her interest into other sensory neuropathies. These conditions are unusual because affected individuals do not feel pain, may not cry tears, and yet may have difficulty with controlling their balance and their blood pressure. Through referral, Felicia has seen several children from Italy with HSAN IV and suggested that they might share a common mutation, although some were clearly less severely affected than others. With the help of Vicki Ciampa (a public affairs leader at NYU) and Roberta Cilio and Claudio Fano (two young neurologists at the Bambino Gesu Hospital in Rome), we set up a study to investigate the mutational basis of HSAN IV. I asked their help with initiating a study of the Roman Jewish community at the same time. Claudio Di Tivoli, the President of the Jewish community, was receptive to their request for help. He invited us into his community and into his home. His small community of 16,000 people is quite illustrious. In his generation, it produced two Nobel Prize winners: the neuroscientist Rita Levi-Montalcini, and Claudio's brother-in-law, economist Federico Modigliani.

Over the course of several days, we recruited people into genetic studies at the Ospedale Bambino Gesu at the Vatican and at the Ospedale Israelitico on the Tiberina Island in Rome—an unusual example of ecumenicalism in the late twentieth century. The Jewish community of Rome is among the oldest, historically continuous Jewish populations. Jews resided in Rome during the Roman Empire and were brought to Rome by the Emperor Titus, following the suppression of the Bar Kochba rebellion and the destruction of the Jewish Temple in Jerusalem in 70 C.E. Spanish Jews came to Rome during the Inquisition and, paradoxically, were shielded from the hostility of their

Roman Jewish neighbors by the Pope. Over time, the Sephardic and Roman Jewish communities co-mingled. Jews from Rome crossed the Alps to populate the Rhine Valley and establish Ashkenazim. So Rome has been a crossroads for Jews from different communities during their histories.

In interviewing more than 100 community members whom we recruited, we learned that most could identify ancestors for at least seven generations and that few had ancestors who had married outside the community in recent times. Many members of the Roman Jewish community were fond of telling us that they were neither Sephardic nor Ashkenazi. Our study from that time demonstrated that the Roman Jews had a low frequency of disease mutations that were found in both Ashkenazi and Sephardic populations, supporting the notion that they may have been a progenitor population for Ashkenazi Jews and that they had Sephardic roots.[191]

Eight years later, I conceived of the Jewish HapMap Project and approached colleagues at Albert Einstein College of Medicine to partner with us in the study. Edward Burns, the Executive Dean, embraced the project and was a prime mover. He worked with me to secure funding from philanthropists and foundations and was often shoulder-to-shoulder with me explaining to people why this project was important to them for understanding their genetic heritage. Much of the early recruitment took place in the Jewish communities of New York.

As the second largest Jewish city in the world, New York was an ideal place to launch the Jewish HapMap Project.

It was not only the size of the population (nearly 2 million) but also the diversity of Jewish Diaspora groups that made the project possible. New York has been a haven for Jewish and other immigrant groups since its founding as New Amsterdam by the Dutch. In his book, *The Island at the Center of World*, Russell Shorto described how the Dutch practice of religious tolerance was brought (somewhat grudgingly) to then New Amsterdam, so that like its namesake in the Netherlands, it was a haven for Sephardic Jews escaping the Inquisition in Brazil.[192] The early wave of Sephardic Jewish immigrants was joined in later generations by Jews from Germany, Eastern Europe, Syria, Iraq, Iran, Central Asia, and other places. The majority of the Ashkenazi Jews came during the great wave of migration of the late nineteenth and early twentieth centuries that brought Fishberg and Jacobs to New York. More recently, with the collapse of the Soviet Union, many Russian Jews have come. The early arrivals, Sephardic and German Jews, have assimilated with their more numerous Ashkenazi Jewish and non-Jewish neighbors. In fact, to recruit Sephardic Jews, Rabbi Marc Angel from the Spanish and Portuguese Synagogue in New York sent me to Seattle, a place where many Turkish and Rhodian (Island of Rhodes) Jews settled during the last century. Yet members of that community also assimilated with more numerous Ashkenazi Jewish neighbors. To recruit even more Sephardic Jews, my Israeli collaborator, Eitan Friedman, and I went to Thessaloniki and Athens, Greece.

The pattern for recruitment was always the same. We always sought support from the rabbinical and lay leadership and the physicians. Often a key person emerged, who aided us with recruitment—among them, Nora Iny and Lana Bakhash from the Iraqi Jewish community, Robert Ohebshalom from the Iranian Jewish community, and Devora Labaton and Robert Matalon from the Syrian Jewish community. These community organizers were important not only for persuading people to participate but also for helping us to improve the design of the study. Robert Ohebshalom hypothesized that the Iranian Jews have a history of geographic isolation in the villages in which they historically resided in Iran, so he made sure that our recruitment included significant representation from those villages. Subsequently, I decided that if we wanted to understand the genetic origins of the whole Jewish Diaspora, we would need to expand our recruitment to other communities in other countries, especially to Israel where many Jewish Diaspora groups went. Eitan Friedman from Sheba Medical Center in Tel Hashomer and David Gurwitz from the National Laboratory for the Genetics of Israeli Populations aided with this effort, especially for recruitment of Moroccan, Algerian, Tunisian, and Libyan Jews from North Africa, Ethiopian, Yemenite, and Indian Jews, and non-Jewish Middle Eastern populations—Druze, Palestinians, and Bedouins. Our analysis team included Li Hao and Alex Pearlman, postdoctoral fellows in my research laboratory; Itsik Pe'er, a computer scientist at Columbia University; his students, Sasha Gunsaev and Pier Francesco Palamara; and

Gil Atzmon, the principal investigator for the project at Albert Einstein College of Medicine.

The Jewish HapMap Project demonstrated in exquisite detail what had been conjectured for a century.[1] Jewish populations from the major Jewish Diaspora groups—Ashkenazi, Sephardic, and Mizrahi—form a distinctive population cluster that is closely related to Semitic and European populations (Figure 4.4). Within this larger Jewish cluster, each of the Jewish populations formed its own subcluster. Each group demonstrated Semitic ancestry and had variable degrees of admixture with European populations. These observations were similar to those of Bonne-Tamir, Cavalli-Sforza, Livshits, Morton, and their coworkers but provided greater precision to their observations and insight into when this occurred.

A high degree of European admixture (30%–60%) was observed among Ashkenazi, Sephardic, Italian, and Syrian Jews (Figure 4.5). As a result, these populations were more closely related to each other than they were to Middle Eastern, Iranian, and Iraqi Jews (Figure 4.6). This genetic split between European/Syrian Jews and Middle Eastern Iraqi and Iranian Jews was timed to have occurred about 2,500 years ago.[28,31,193] The European and Syrian Jewish populations were formed over the last 2,000 years by people who migrated from or were expelled from Palestine and by individuals who were converted to Judaism when proselytism was commonplace during Hellenic-Hasmonean times. Religious proscriptions about marrying non-Jews during the past 2,000 years in

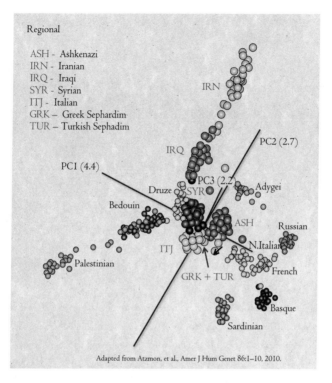

Regional

ASH - Ashkenazi
IRN - Iranian
IRQ - Iraqi
SYR - Syrian
ITJ - Italian
GRK — Greek Sephardim
TUR — Turkish Sephadim

IRN

PC2 (2.7)

IRQ

PCI (4.4)

PC3 (2.2)
Druze   SYR   Adygei

Bedouin

ASH   Russian

Palestinian   ITJ   N.Italia

GRK + TUR   French

Basque

Sardinian

Adapted from Atzmon, et al., Amer J Hum Genet 86:1–10, 2010.

Figure 4.4. Principle component analysis demonstrating that Ashkenazi, Sephardic, and Mizrahi Jews form a distinctive population cluster that is closely related to Middle Eastern non-Jewish and European populations. Within this larger cluster, each of the Jewish populations forms its own subcluster. (See color figure.)

all of these Diaspora Jewish groups made recent large-scale admixture unlikely. Yet, these observations did not exclude cumulative low-level admixture with neighboring non-Jewish communities. These observations also refuted the theories that Ashkenazi Jews are the descendants of converted Khazars or Slavs.[36,134]

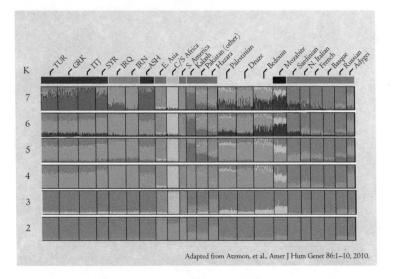

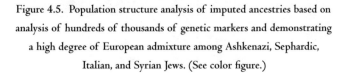

Adapted from Atzmon, et al., Amer J Hum Genet 86:1–10, 2010.

Figure 4.5. Population structure analysis of imputed ancestries based on analysis of hundreds of thousands of genetic markers and demonstrating a high degree of European admixture among Ashkenazi, Sephardic, Italian, and Syrian Jews. (See color figure.)

Our analyses showed that the Sephardic Jews of Greece and Turkey were almost indistinguishable from one another, having common ancestry from emigrating Sephardic Jews from Spain and Portugal who admixed over time with Romaniote Jews of the Byzantine Empire. Large-scale admixture between Sephardic Jews from Spain and Portugal following the Spanish Inquisition with the Jews of Syria may have accounted for the genetic closeness that we observed between Syrian Jews with Turkish and Greek Jews. Significant admixture between Sephardic and Ashkenazi Jews has been reported, especially in Bulgaria and

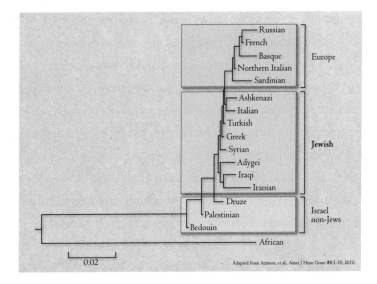

Figure 4.6. Neighbor joining tree demonstrating genetic sharing among
Jewish groups and a split between European/Syrian Jews and Middle
Eastern Iraqi and Iranian Jews that was timed to have occurred
approximately 2500 years ago. (See color figure.)

Romania, historically transitional zones between the Austro-
Hungarian and Ottoman empires. This may have contributed
to the genetic proximity of Sephardic and Ashkenazi Jewish
populations[31,144] and has been observed in mitochondrial haplogroups shared by Bulgarian and Ashkenazi Jews.[144]

The results for the Italians Jews from Rome were concor-
dant with their claim to be neither Ashkenazi nor Sephardic
Jewish.[194] The proximity of these Roman Jews to both
Ashkenazi and Sephardic Jews supported the notion that they

may have been progenitors to Ashkenazi Jews and that both Ashkenazi and Sephardic Jews later admixed with Roman Jews. The Iranian and Iraqi Jews formed their own relatively large clusters with the greatest genetic distances from the other populations and the least distances from each other. The divergence of these groups following the Babylonian exile provided more time for accumulation of genetic diversity. The greater differentiation of Iranian and Iraqi Jews might also be explained on the basis of local marriages, which are frequently consanguineous and often within a certain social class or with a certain social structure. In addition to the Southern Europeans, the closest genetic neighbors to most Jewish groups were the Palestinians, Israeli Bedouins, and Druze. The genetic clusters formed by each of these non-Jewish Middle Eastern groups reflects their own histories of marrying within the group.[195–197] Their proximity to one another and to European and Syrian Jews suggested a shared genetic history of related Semitic and non-Semitic Mediterranean ancestors who chose different religious and tribal affiliations. Rosenberg's earlier study of Israeli Jewish, Palestinian, and Druze populations made a similar observation by demonstrating the proximity of these two non-Jewish populations to Ashkenazi and Iraqi Jews.[180] The Jewish HapMap Project showed that the Jewish people in the populations studied represent a series of geographical isolates or clusters woven together by common genetic threads.

Within the Jewish HapMap Project, these threads were observed as strands of DNA that were identical between individuals both within specific Diaspora Jewish populations and among populations, demonstrating shared ancestry. Jewish populations shared more and longer segments with one another than with non-Jewish populations, highlighting the commonality of Jewish origin. The degree of sharing was highest among Iranian and Iraqi Jews and less so among Turkish and Greek Jews, reflecting a higher degree of marrying within the family, or endogamy—a practice that was common in Middle Eastern communities. Overall, the typical degree of sharing was what might be expected for fourth or fifth cousins; this, indeed, is the degree of relatedness within Jewish communities. Unlike the other populations, the Ashkenazi Jews exhibited increased sharing of segments at the shorter end of the range but decreased sharing at the longer end. This pattern in which older shared segments got shorter and few new ones were created is consistent with a population bottleneck followed by rapid expansion. This corresponded to the so-called *demographic miracle* of Ashkenazi Jewish history in which the population expanded from 50,000 people at the beginning of the fifteenth century to 5 million people at the beginning of the nineteenth century.[33]

Shortly after our study was published, a study was published by Behar, Skorecki, Villems, and their collaborators that included populations that we had not analyzed.[4] They noted the same clustering of Jewish populations that we had observed. This cluster included North African and Central Asian but not Ethiopian (Beta Israel) nor Indian (B'nei Israel and Cochini) Jewish populations. This work also demonstrated that the

Jewish populations within the shared cluster traced their origins in part to the Middle East.

Since then, our team completed a study of North African Jewish groups (Moroccan, Algerian, Tunisian, Djerban, and Libyan) that demonstrated distinctive clusters that were, nonetheless, part of a larger Ashkenazi and Sephardic Jewish group. These North African Jews had variable degrees of Middle Eastern, European, and North African ancestry, yet were quite different from contemporary populations from North and South Morocco, Western Sahara, Tunisia, Libya, and Egypt. Two major subgroups were identified—Moroccan/Algerian Jews and Djerban/Libyan Jews that varied in their degree of European admixture. These genetic analyses showed that members of these North African Jewish groups had married within their ranks over long periods of time—akin to what Rosenberg had described earlier for Libyan Jews. Together, these studies demonstrated that the history of the Jewish Diasporas could be seen in the genomes of Jewish people—founding during Classical Antiquity with proselytism of local populations, followed by genetic isolation with the rise of Christianity and then Islam, and admixture in some groups following the emigration of Sephardic Jews during the Inquisition.

FIVE

TRAITS

More than a century ago, Francis Galton, the famous English polymath, wrote *Hereditary Genius*, a book that captured the public's attention (Figure 5.1).[198] Interest in this topic has not vanished with time. Galton argued that superior intelligence tends to be transmitted within families. Is this because intelligent parents nurture intelligence in their offspring? Galton thought not. He tried to show that "a man's natural abilities are derived by inheritance." He believed that it would be "quite practicable to produce a highly gifted race of men by judicious marriages during several, consecutive generations." Galton examined clustering of professions within families and acknowledged that nepotism could play as important a role as intelligence for forming such clusters. Yet, in his

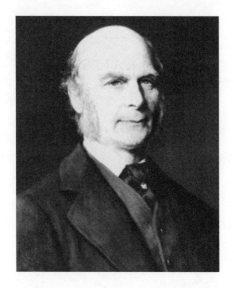

Figure 5.1. Photo of Sir Frances Galton, English polymath, who was
an advocate for measuring human traits. His book, *Hereditary Genius*,
spawned the Nature versus Nurture debate that lingers to today.

view, nepotism could not account for clustering of high-quality
reputations—only heredity could.

Galton was influenced by the writing of his cousin, Charles
Darwin, who showed in his book, *The Variation of Animals and Plants
under Domestication*, that selection for superior traits can occur
through breeding in animals or plants.[199] Although Galton studied intellectual ability in selected English families, he noted that
he would have liked "to investigate the biographies of Italians
and Jews, both of whom appear to be rich in families of high
intellectual breeds."[198] Galton's affinity for Jews was both shared
and reviled by his contemporaries and successors.

Galton's protégé, Joseph Jacobs, acted upon Galton's interest by studying the biographies of European Jews to produce a list of distinguished people.[200] After applying some *corrections*, he determined that "there is about twice as much chance of finding a distinguished man among Jews as among Englishmen." Jacobs' list contained the names of many men and women of Jewish origin who had been raised Christian or had converted to Christianity. This list included the names of people, such as Karl Marx, Benjamin Disraeli, Heinrich Heine, and Felix Mendelssohn, whose eminence has withstood the test of time. It also included the names of some lesser luminaries, such as Berthold Auerbach ("Germany's greatest novelist"), Theodor Benfey ("the greatest philologist in Germany"), Abraham Geiger ("the head of the Jewish Reform movement"), and Heinreich Graetz ("the Jewish Macaulay"), who are less likely to be known widely. In producing the list, Jacobs corrected for the underrepresentation of Russian and Rumanian Jews, who lived in countries that were repressive of their large Jewish populations and limited possibilities for achieving eminence. He found that Jewish men tended to excel in music, mathematics, metaphysics, linguistics, and finance and noted, "Equally striking is the comparatively large number of Jewesses (Jewish women), no less than thirteen, figuring there as actresses, writers, or leaders of salons." Jacobs also placed some caveats, noting that his work, "which puts Jewish ability in a favourable light, emanates from a Jew." To guard against the possible imputation that his work represented "bad taste" or "bad science," Jacobs vowed that he was conscious of being biased toward Jews in the process of performing his study.

The issue of Jews and intelligence has resurfaced many times since Jacobs' and Galton's era. In 1928, A.G. Hughes published a study of schoolchildren in the *Eugenics Review* that demonstrated "the innate superiority of London Jewish schoolchildren over their Gentile schoolmates."[201] Hughes noted, "That Jews differ from non-Jews is generally accepted as an axiomatic truth, but that most of the descriptions of such differences are based on unscientific observations heavily biased by strong feelings." This study of psychometric test performance was undertaken by Dr. Cyril Burt and Miss Mary Davies in three London schools, representative of three levels of social and economic status and each with sizable numbers of Jewish and non-Jewish students. The children were given the Northumberland Standardized Tests in Generalized Intelligence, Arithmetic, and English, and mental ages were compared—"mental age" was determined as the average score for children of a certain chronological age. At each school, the Jewish children outperformed their non-Jewish classmates: their mental ages were roughly a year ahead in every case. Jewish boys and girls both had higher mental ages than their age-matched peers. A gradient in performance was observed for socio-economic status. Jews and non-Jews alike were approximately a year ahead at the best schools and a year behind at the worst. This correlation between performance and socio-economic status held up when parent's profession, rather than location of the school, was compared. Hughes was careful to qualify his observations. He pointed out that the differences might be more apparent than real and that the non-Jewish children would catch up to their Jewish classmates in time. He also pointed out that these observations might be applicable only to Jews then living in London but not to Jews living in other places and other times. Nonetheless, he restated Galton's argument that "the Jewish superiority is not temporary; rather it is the result of generations of 'breeding for intelligence.'"

But were his observations true? In 1974, Princeton psychologist Leon Kamin noted that when Burt increased his sample size for identical twins reared apart from fewer than 20 to more than 50, the average correlation for IQ between pairs remained the same to the third decimal place—that is, Kamin assumed that Burt's analysis of his data was too good to be true and must have been fudged.[202] (It should be noted that in the twentiethth century, Mendel was charged with having fudged his data because the distribution was too good to be true.[203]) Later, in 1976, London *Sunday Times* medical correspondent Oliver Gillie observed that two of Burt's supposed collaborators, people who allegedly collected and processed his data, never existed at all.[204] These criticisms were enshrined in *The Mismeasure of Man*, Stephen Jay Gould's Pulitzer Prize-winning book about the fallacies of psychometric testing to measure intelligence.[205] He noted, "The intense debate about Cyril Burt's later work has focused exclusively on the fakery of his late career. This perspective clouded Sir Cyril's greater influence as the most powerful mental tester committed to a factor-analytic model of intelligence as a real and unitary 'thing'". Burt was convinced that intelligence was a unitary thing (in the parlance of geneticists, a "phenotype") that was determined by heritable factors ("genes"). Indeed, refutation of this point-of-view forms the central argument against a genetic basis for intelligence and its proxy, IQ. If it is not a real and unitary thing, then it cannot be genetically determined. This argument has continued to be played out up to the present.

In 2007, Charles Murray, the conservative political analyst, published an article in *Commentary Magazine* called "Jewish Genius"—a play on words from Galton's "Hereditary Genius."[206] Murray and Herrnstein's work, *The Bell Curve*, was one of the most controversial books of the 1990s, because they espoused the notion debated by Gould and others that there was a unitary intelligence that could be measured by IQ testing.[207] Murray and Herrnstein outraged their detractors and the public by espousing the notion that IQ was in part genetically determined, and like Garod and Jacobs, they believed that the median and range of IQs varied among ethnic groups. This book stirred the pot of the nature versus nurture intelligence debate. They noted, "Large human populations differ in many ways, both cultural and biological. It is not surprising that they might differ at least slightly in their characteristics." They went on to state, "Jews—specifically Ashkenazi Jews of European origins—test higher than any other ethnic group. The literature indicates that Jews in America and Britain have an overall IQ mean somewhere between a half and a full standard deviation

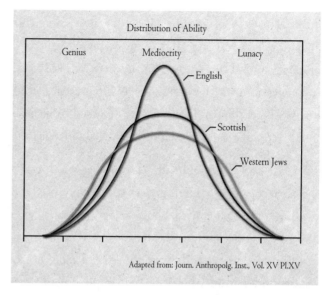

Figure 5.2. Joseph Jacobs' observations about IQ distributions in different populations, allegedly demonstrating a higher proportion of "genius" and "lunacy" among Scots and Jews. (See color figure.)

above the mean, with the source of the difference concentrated in the verbal component."[207–208] The premise included the idea that, if the bell curve of intelligence was skewed toward having a higher mean for IQ, then a larger number of individuals at the higher end would fall into the genius range (Figure 5.2; notably, Jacobs presented his data in a similar fashion more than a century earlier). Cochran, Hardy, and Harpending quantified the magnitude of this effect.

While the mean IQ difference between Ashkenazim and other northern Europeans may not seem large, such a small difference maps to a large difference in the proportion of the population with very high IQs...For example, if the mean Ashkenazi IQ is 110 and the standard deviation is 15, then the number of northern Europeans with IQs greater than 140 should be 4 per thousand while 23 per thousand Ashkenazim should exceed the same threshold – a six-fold difference.[208]

Some 15 years after publishing *The Bell Curve*, Murray revisited the issue of Jewish intelligence, specifically at the upper end of the curve. Murray, a Scots-Irish Quaker from Iowa, proved to be a Judeophile. Like Jacobs, he was impressed by Jewish accomplishment. In his article, *Jewish Genius*, he covered the timing and nature of Jewish accomplishment, focusing on the arts and sciences and picking up where Jacobs left off. From 1870 to 1950, Jewish representation in literature was four times the number one would expect; in music and visual arts, five times; in chemistry, six times; and so forth. In the first half of the twentieth century, Jews won 14% of Nobel Prizes in literature, chemistry, physics, and medicine/physiology. In the second half of the twentieth century, that figure rose to 29%. Murray believed that Jews were not only *nurtured* to be smart, but also they were *bred* to be smart.

Murray had an explanation for the recent occurrence of Jewish accomplishment—the potential was always there. It took lifting the impediments for the potential to be realized. He noted:

> The sparse representation of Jews during the flowering of the European arts and sciences is not hard to explain.

They were systematically excluded, both by legal restrictions on the occupations they could enter and by savage social discrimination. Then came legal emancipation, beginning in the late 1700s in a few countries and completed in Western Europe by the 1870s, and with it one of the most extraordinary stories of any ethnic group at any point in human history. As soon as Jewish children born under legal emancipation had time to grow to adulthood, they started appearing in the first ranks of the arts and sciences. During the four decades from 1830 to 1870, when the first Jews to live under emancipation reached their forties, 16 significant Jewish figures appear. In the next four decades, from 1870 to 1910, the number jumps to 40.

In this article, Murray put himself out on a speculative limb for why the latent Jewish potential for accomplishment developed. "Two potential explanations for a Jewish gene pool favoring high intelligence are so obvious that many people assume they must be true: winnowing by persecution (only the smartest Jews either survived or remained Jews) and marrying for brains (scholars and children of scholars were socially desirable spouses). Murray was supported in his perspective on discrimination as a selective force by earlier writers. Albert Einstein wrote, "It may be thanks to anti-Semitism that we are able to preserve our race,"[209] and Isaac Bashevis Singer, the Nobel Prize-winning Jewish writer, wrote, "It is the good fortune of the Jewish people that for 2000 years they didn't have any power. The little bit of power that they did have they have certainly misused like anyone else who has power."[210] As noted in Chapter 4, evidence for selective mating is readily observed in the genomes of Jewish peoples and for a bottleneck, which was followed by rapid expansion, that can be observed in the genomes of Ashkenazi Jewish people; but neither of these is "proof" for Murray's arguments.

Murray was surprised that Jews were reluctant to address the issue of Jewish accomplishment themselves. He pointed out, "*Commentary* has never published a systematic discussion of one of the most obvious topics of all: the extravagant overrepresentation of Jews, relative to their numbers, in the top ranks of the arts, sciences, law, medicine, finance, entrepreneurship, and the media."[206] He went on to note:

> I have personal experience with the reluctance of Jews to talk about Jewish accomplishment—my coauthor, the late Richard Herrnstein, gently resisted the paragraphs on Jewish IQ that I insisted on putting in *The Bell Curve* (1994). Both history and the contemporary revival of anti-Semitism in Europe make it easy to understand the reasons for that reluctance.

Going out farther on a speculative limb, Cochran, Hardy, and Harpending linked selection for intelligence with selection for genetic disease genes. They suggested that selection accounted for the high frequency of carriers for lysosomal storage diseases, such as Gaucher and Tay-Sachs, and that the altered biochemical properties of neurons of mutation carriers provided the basis for enhanced Ashkenazi Jewish intelligence. Contemporary geneticists have not embraced this theory because they view the evidence as flimsy and circumstantial. Quoting UCSF geneticist Neil Risch, in her *New York Magazine* article about this paper, writer Jennifer Senior noted, "The authors' hypothesis that what's being selected for is intelligence is a sexy guess, it's based on almost nothing concrete."[211] Building on this critical assessment, Risch stated, "Jews have been accused of being frugal, cheap, aggressive. There's a clear survival advantage to those traits too. Why not pick on those?"

Although published reports provide support for an IQ differential among Ashkenazi Jews residing not only in the United States and London but also in Israel, a study of Israeli children provided a clue for what may actually be occurring. In 1967, Ortar summarized the experience with 12 years of achievement testing of Israeli eighth graders.[212] From 1955 to 1967, every student in the eighth grade of Israeli primary schools took a test to determine who would be eligible for a grant to attend secondary school. Ortar was the inspector in the Israeli Ministry of Culture and Education who was entrusted with the yearly task of compiling the results and making suggestions for possible modifications. She found the problem particularly perplexing because the school achievement for half of the students in her survey was inadequate. She observed a divide in performance between the Ashkenazi Jewish students (called "European") and the non-Ashkenazi Jewish students (called "Oriental"). The Israeli-born children of

"Oriental-born" parents scored lower on these tests than did their peers who were born to "European-born" parents, but the test results changed over time. This scoring gap improved in the next generation of children born to Israeli-born parents.

This observation of a performance gap between Ashkenazi and non-Ashkenazi Jews might have been construed as evidence of an innate intellectual endowment for Ashkenazi Jews, the Israeli equivalent of *The Bell Curve*. In fact, it is a typical manifestation of what has become known as the *Flynn Effect*. This effect is named for James Flynn, a Professor of Political Studies at the University of Otago in New Zealand. He demonstrated in the 1980s that mean IQ scores changed by 5 to 25 points in a single generation, indicating that it is not a stable measure of innate intelligence. Flynn has written, "About 1981, it struck me that if IQ gains over time had occurred anywhere, they might have occurred everywhere and that a phenomenon of great significance was being overlooked. Therefore I began to survey to see what data existed throughout the developed world."[213] Rather, the changes in IQ scores reflect changes in learning. Gains in education are leading to gains in IQ performance. Second-generation Israelis do not have a genetic makeup that differs from their parents or grandparents. Rather, they have been acculturated into Israeli society and have learned how to take the standardized tests.

But the Flynn Effect was known even before it was discovered by Flynn. Writing in *The Bell Curve Wars*, Sowell has noted, "Mental test results from American soldiers tested in

World War II showed that their performances on these tests
were higher than the performances of American soldiers in
World War I by the equivalent of about twelve IQ points."[214]
He went on to state:

> Perhaps the most dramatic changes were those in the mental
> test performances of Jews in the United States. The results
> of World War I mental tests conducted among American
> soldiers born in Russia — the great majority of whom were
> Jews — showed such low scores as to cause Carl Bingham,
> creator of the Scholastic Aptitude Test, to declare that
> these results "disprove the popular belief that the Jew is
> highly intelligent."

The temporal changes in IQ that Sowell described among
Ashkenazi Jews in the United States and that Ortar described
among Oriental Jews in Israel have occurred many times over
the past 200 years for Jews living in diverse locales. These
resulted from access to education and legal emancipation. One
Iranian Jewish physician described this to me quite well during
the process of recruitment for the Jewish HapMap Project.
He stated, "Previously we were poor and lived in villages and
were barely literate. When the *Alliance* schools opened, we were
able to get a primary and secondary education and then go
to the University of Teheran where we excelled, and became
professionals." The other benefits that his family gained in the
twentieth century were citizenship and equal rights before the
law. Remarkably, the Jews gained full rights during the reign

of Reza Shah Pahlevi, the father of the last shah of Iran. The resulting economic success of Iranian Jews has rivaled that of Ashkenazi Jews.

One of the lynchpins to the economic and intellectual betterment of North African and Middle Eastern Jews was the *Alliance Israelite Universelle*. The *Alliance* was founded in Paris in 1860 to promote the rights of Jews throughout the world and to defend them from persecution. The founders were imbued with the liberal ideas that had emanated from the French Revolution and from the Napoleonic Era. They thought that the emancipation of Jews with the granting of equal rights and full citizenship was destined to spread throughout the world and to transform all Jewish communities. They believed, "All Jews are responsible for each other," but also that Jews themselves had to change if they were to merit emancipation. As Rodrigue has written, "They had to transform themselves into enlightened, modern citizens, abandoning their peculiaristic habits and attitudes…In the classic terminology of the Enlightenment, the Jews had to be 'regenerated' in order to show themselves worthy of emancipation and citizenship."[215]

To effect this regeneration, the *Alliance* created a vast network of schools in the Middle East and North Africa, stretching from Morocco to Iran. The Muslim powers generally did not offer much resistance to the establishment of French-language schools. Although similar in scope to French governmental efforts to promote French political influence, language, and culture, the *Alliance* was an independent, nongovernmental organization. It maintained its independence by having an international membership that paid an annual subscription fee. Its activities were subsidized by the Baron Maurice de Hirsch and his wife. In addition to academic and religious instruction, some of the schools developed apprenticeship programs to train their students for the trades. At its peak in 1914, 43,700 students were attending 183 Alliance schools.[216] The reach of the *Alliance* was incomplete, as observed by Ortar's study of the children of North African and Middle Eastern Jewish immigrants. Where it succeeded on its own terms, the effects were quite dramatic—as food writer Claudia Roden noted when describing her upbringing in Cairo:

> The Egypt I knew was a French-speaking cosmopolitan country in which life for the better-off was a sort of continuation of the Belle Époque in an annex of Europe…The Jewish community had a happy and important place in the mosaic of minorities—which included Copts, Armenians, Syrian Christians, Maltese, Greeks, and Italians, as well as British and French expatriates—living among the Moslem majority.[217]

So breeding, selection, and education may all have contributed to Jewish intellectual accomplishment, but so, too, did being in the right place at the right time. In his book, *Outliers*, Gladwell added the new element of Jewish opportunities to the mix of Jewish genes, Jewish mothers, and Jewish schools.[218] In his chapter on powerhouse New York Jewish lawyers, Gladwell made the point that all were born around 1930. As a result, they came of age during a Depression Era demographic drought, when fewer kids in schools got more time from teachers. They went on to good colleges and good law schools. When they graduated, for the most part they were kept out of New York City white-shoe WASP law firms, because of the anti-Semitic snobbery during the 1950s. As a result, they started their own firms. These have become the powerhouse firms of today, because these lawyers turned to areas of the law like stock proxy fights and hostile takeover bids, which were unglamorous in the 1950s but extremely remunerative in the 1970s and 1980s. So their accidents of birth and standing as young lawyers gave them the greatest of opportunities. In a subchapter of *Outliers*, Gladwell called their accidents of birth and standing, "The Importance of Being Jewish."

Being in the right place at the right time also impacted the great success of the Hungarian Jewish physicists of the 1930s and 1940s, although their accidents of birth and standing were quite different. Rather than having humble origins, theirs were quite illustrious. In the turn-of-the-century Hungary, the 850,000 Jews comprised only 5% of the population but were the leaders of capitalism and industry.[219] By 1910, they comprised more than 50% of Hungary's lawyers, commercial businessmen, and physicians and 80% of the country's financiers. Their roles in the economic boom in Hungary made them very wealthy. By the start of World War I, 346 Hungarian Jewish families had been given aristocratic titles by the emperor. Out of this exceptional Hungarian Jewish middle class came

seven of the twentieth century's most illustrious physicists—
Theodore von Kármán, George de Hevesy, Michael Polanyi,
Leó Szilárd, Eugene Wigner, John von Neumann, and Edward
Teller. Two of the seven, de Hevesy and Wigner, won Nobel
Prizes. Frits Houtermans, a theoretical physicist, proposed
jokingly that these people, "were really visitors from Mars; for
them, it was difficult to speak without an accent that would
give them away and therefore they chose to pretend to be
Hungarians whose inability to speak any language without an
accent is well-known."

Yet accidents of birth, wealth, privilege, and education are
not sufficient to explain who will become outstanding lawyers
or physicists. The historian of science, Derek de Solla Price,
provided another reason in his book, Little Science, Big Science.[220]
Reworking Galton's data and other, similar datasets, he noted,
"We now know that the total number of scientists goes up as the
square, more or less, of the number of good ones. Therefore, if
we want to multiply the good scientists by 5, we must multiply
the whole group by 25." He reasoned that a certain threshold
of intelligence was required for being a (little) scientist and that
the good (big) scientists markedly exceeded this threshold and,
perhaps, had a threshold of their own. Given the Gaussian (bell
curve) distribution of intelligence, significantly fewer scientists
would surpass the upper threshold required for being a good
scientist than the threshold for being a scientist. This same line
of reasoning was adopted by Murray more than a quarter of a
century later to explain the distribution of intelligence in the

Ashkenazi Jewish population and the skew in all IQ scores that generated more Nobel Prize winners. He stated:

> A group's mean intelligence is important in explaining outcomes, such as mean educational attainment or mean income. The key indicator for predicting *exceptional* accomplishment (like winning a Nobel Prize) is the incidence of exceptional intelligence. Consider an IQ score of 140 or higher, denoting the level of intelligence that can permit people to excel in fields like theoretical physics and pure mathematics. If the mean Jewish IQ is 110 and the standard deviation is 15, then the proportion of Jews with IQs of 140 or higher is somewhere around six times the proportion of everyone else.

Hungarian Jews in the 1930s and 1940s and American Jews at mid-century may have been years ahead in the Flynn Effect, waiting for others to catch up. Or their early-onset Flynn Effect may have been genetically endowed. Both groups had the good fortune of being born at the right time and place for investigating contemporary physics and practicing corporate law. Still, as Gladwell has pointed out in *Outliers,* no single factor is completely predictive of any individual's success within a given realm.

Despite much criticism, the notion that general intelligence and its proxy, IQ, are genetically determined has not faded. The assumption of a heritable basis for IQ and for other traits has come from studies of identical twins reared together and apart. The value of studying twins for sorting genetic and environmental effects has been appreciated since Galton published his paper, "The history of twins, as a criterion of the relative power of nature and nurture," in 1876.[221] Gould wrote:

> If I had any desire to lead a life of indolent ease, I would wish to be an identical twin, separated from my brother at birth and reared in a different social class. We could hire ourselves out to a host of social scientists and practically name our fee. For we would be exceedingly rarer representatives of the only really adequate natural experiment for separating genetic from environmental affecting humans – genetically identical individuals raised in disparate environment.[205]

From comparing the close similarity of IQ scores for identical twins reared apart (who share genes but not an environment) to twins reared together (who share both), it has been possible to estimate how much of the variation in IQ and other traits can be accounted for by genetic factors. Psychologist Ian Dreary and his coworkers have written:

> The g factor is among the most replicated findings in psychology…Lest people wonder whether g factors extracted from different assemblages of mental tests would differ—and therefore might rank people quite differently—it has been demonstrated that, when test batteries are even reasonably diverse, g scores from different batteries of tests correlate all-but perfectly.[214]

University of Pittsburgh computational geneticist Bernie Devlin and her Carnegie-Melon colleagues Kathryn Roeder and

Michael Daniels analyzed data from 212 different studies, such as the Swedish Adoption/Twin Study of Aging, and determined that the heritability of IQ was 0.48—that is, about half of the variance in IQ scores could be explained by genetic factors. Other studies have estimated the heritability to be between 0.40 and 0.80.[214] Heritabilities for other traits have been quantified that are higher (height 0.8), similar (weight 0.5), or lower (systolic blood pressure 0.3, birth weight 0.1).

So despite arguments for the reification of the Flynn Effect and against the reification of IQ, studies are being conducted to identify genetic markers that are predictive of IQ. Perhaps the most robust of these studies was a genome-wide association study, or GWAS.[222] The GWAS was the direct beneficiary of the International HapMap Project, because that project identified millions of genetic markers that could be used to identify the genes that predispose to virtually any human trait. One of our major reasons for undertaking the Jewish HapMap Project was to develop maps saturated with genetic markers for Jewish populations that could be used to identify the genes that predispose to virtually any human trait in Jews. GWAS now use DNA chips with 1,000,000 or more markers (or SNPs) scattered across the genome. The development of this chip-based technology was itself as important as the HapMap for facilitating GWAS. In a typical study, hundreds, thousands, or even more individuals are analyzed for a specific trait. Studies with so many subjects and so many markers have many confounders that create confusion, generating large numbers of false–positive results.

As noted, one of the major confounders is mismatching of cases and controls for ancestry. A study enriched for Ashkenazi Jewish cases and non-Jewish European controls will identify markers that are predictive of ancestry, rather than the trait in question. Because differences in ancestry can be discerned precisely using many genetic markers, ancestry analysis is now built into such studies, and statistical methods are applied to correct for a possible mismatch. To correct for the spurious associations that may occur by chance alone when large numbers of comparisons are being made, the threshold for calling a significant association is set very low. The commonly used metric for measuring statistical significance is the p-value. The common threshold of significance, a p-value of 0.05, indicates that a similar result could be obtained by chance alone 1 in 20 times. Applying a p-value of 0.05 in a GWAS means that for a DNA chip with 1,000,000 SNPs, a positive result would be obtained for 50,000 markers on the basis of chance alone. To lessen the possibility for such spurious results, the threshold is established at 1 in 100 million or possibly even lower.

GWAS have been performed now for hundreds of different traits. These have identified SNPs that influence blood pressure, breast cancer, height, and many other traits, including IQ. A striking feature of these efforts is that one study tends to replicate another. When the results are pooled across studies, p-values as small as one in a hundred trillion and even less have been observed. The probabilities of these associations are too small to have occurred by chance alone. GWAS of these traits have shown that SNPs in multiple genes—often in pathways of genes that are known to work together—influence the development of a trait. The magnitude of the effect of a given SNP may be large, but more often, it is slight and accounts for only a small effect on the trait in question.

To date, only one sizeable GWAS was performed for general cognitive ability (g).[223] This study was performed by Robert Plomin, an American psychologist who lives and works in London, and his associates. Plomin's research focuses on identical twins reared together or apart, the very representatives Gould noted in the natural experiment for separating genetic from environmental effects in humans. The GWAS was performed on 7-year-olds from Plomin's Twins Early Development Study of nearly 11,000 twins born in Great Britain in the early 1990s. Four standardized verbal and nonverbal tests were administered to the children over the phone, and the scores on each of the individual tests were added to create a measure of g. One of the twins was selected for inclusion in the genetic analysis. The study was performed in two stages, using a study design that has been used in other GWAS. In the first stage, equal amounts of DNA were pooled for children in one of two groups—one with average g and the other with high g. The average g group was comprised of 458 children and the high g group of 420 children, each with approximately equal numbers of boys and girls. In the second stage, an independent sample of 3,195 children representative of the entire group of 7,000 7-year-olds were tested for the 47 SNPs that were found to be significant in the first stage. Six of these SNPs were replicated in the second study, producing a similar result for demonstrating significant genetic association with g. The genetic effect was small. None of these SNPs accounted for more than 0.4% of this effect. Furthermore, none of the SNPs was in a gene that might have been predicted to be associated with intelligence. Surprising though this may seem, it is in keeping with the discoveries of other GWAS, where novel genes have been identified that might not have been predicted prior to the study. This small effect size for each of these genes was similar to the small effects observed for genetic determinants of weight and height with variants in many genes contributing the effect.

This is the first of many such studies that might be anticipated. In fact, there is much work to be done to identify the genetic variants that account for the high heritability of intelligence defined by Devlin and others. In these future studies, the results of some of these six markers will be replicated, new markers will be identified, the prevalence of these markers will be found to vary in different populations, and new theories will be formulated to explain the effect of the SNPs on cognitive function. These studies will be complemented by sequencing whole genomes to identify not only SNPs, but also rare genetic variants, that influence intelligence. Some investigators may even try to formulate that the prevalence of certain advantageous SNPs or rare genetic variants contributes to the perceived intellectual advantages of a specific ethnic group. Clearly, the work to date suggests that the intellectual accomplishments of Jewish people have been determined not only by the group from which they came but also by the circumstances of that group, often being in the right or wrong place at a given time in history.

An issue of even greater contention is that of genetics and mental illness. In the early twentieth century, Fishberg expressed this issue in fairly quaint terms, "The fact that Jews in every country are more liable to mental derangement than their non-Jewish neighbors would speak in favour of racial peculiarity in this respect."[8] Fishberg provided both nature and nurture arguments to explain this increased frequency—the complexity of modern life, the marriage of near kin, urbanization. Goodman combed the medical literature of his time and came to the opposite conclusion, when he observed, "What once seemed certain in the minds of many—that the rate of mental illness is extremely high [in Jews]—can no longer be accepted as a truism."[63]

This issue has lingered since Goodman's time. Brown University psychiatrist Robert Kohn reviewed the medical literature about mental illness in Jews and wrote in 1994 that Ashkenazi Jews have higher rates of manic-depressive disorders than Sephardic or North African Jews but felt that these studies were all flawed by a greater tendency among Ashkenazi Jews to seek psychiatric help. They were also complicated by unreliability in diagnoses and failure to account for differences in social class, immigration status, and exposure to the Holocaust—all factors that might have affected the apparent frequency of mental illness.[224] Kohn and his coworkers then went on to investigate the frequency of mental illness among Israeli Jews using a study design that was not based on seeking psychiatric help. Their approach involved use of a structured interview searching for psychiatric symptoms among a cohort of almost 5,000 24- to 38-year-old Israeli-born offspring of immigrants. This study yielded a different result from the first—the North African Jews had a higher frequency of intermittent and severe depression, whereas the Ashkenazi Jews had a higher frequency of manic episodes.[225] Kohn participated in a similar study in the United States, the Epidemiologic Catchment Area (ECA) program of the National Institute of Mental Health.[226] This study was undertaken to determine the prevalence and incidence of mental disorders and on the use of and need for services by the mentally ill. This study also used a structured interview format that was undertaken three times over the course of a year. The study was performed at five sites across the United States. At each site, more than 3,000 community residents and 500 residents of institutions were sampled, yielding 20,861 respondents overall. Mental illness diagnoses were made using a manual that provided specific criteria, the *Diagnostic and Statistical Manual of Mental Disorders*, then in its third edition (DSM-III). Kohn's group of investigators compared Jews with non-Jews (e.g., Protestants, Catholics, atheists, and others) in New Haven, Connecticut, and Los Angeles, California, where the Jews comprised approximately 9% of the total group at those sites. Two findings stood out from their study. The Jewish men had a higher rate of major depression than their non-Jewish male counterparts; thus, the rate of major depression was similar between Jewish men and Jewish women. As a result, the rate of depression among Jewish women was no different from their non-Jewish female counterparts. Yet, geneticists working today seem to share Goodman's point-of-view that the rates of mild or severe manic-depressive disease do not differ between Jews and non-Jews.[227]

That mental illness can have a genetic basis has been long suspected. In a study of the Finnish Twin Cohort, the heritability of bipolar I disorder (the most severe form) was estimated to be 93%.[228] High heritabilities of bipolar disease have been observed in twin cohorts in the Denmark, Norway, Sweden, and the United Kingdom as have the most devastating consequence of this illness—suicide.[229] Alec Roy, a psychiatrist at the Veterans Administration Hospital in New Jersey, counted 400 pedigrees in the medical literature in which at least one of the twins committed suicide. Of the 129 identical twin pairs, 17 committed suicide. Of the 270 fraternal twin pairs, only 2 did—again an instance of high heritability.[230] Even before these cohorts of twins were studied, individual cases of twin suicides were reported. Kay Redfield Jamison, a professor of psychiatry at Johns Hopkins University School of Medicine and herself afflicted with manic depressive disease, has become our foremost chronicler of this disorder. In her book on understanding suicide, *Night Falls Fast*, Jameson wrote about Captains CL and JL, identical twins who served honorably in the Revolutionary War.[231] Within a few years of each other following the war, both committed suicide after a period of melancholy. Jamison reported not only about twins but also about other families with clusters of individuals who committed suicide. The most notable of these was the Briggs family, which counted more than 20 suicides during a period of more than 50 years, leaving them with no survivors.

Jamison has also described studies of family members who are reared apart, because:

> The findings from the twin studies provide strong evidence for a genetic effect, but family dynamics and psychological issues inevitably confound their interpretation. One way of further isolating environmental from genetic influences is by conducting an adoption study. Individuals who are adopted share their genes, but not their environment, with their biological parents; conversely, they share their environment, but no genes, with their adoptive parents. Adoption therefore creates a unique natural experiment.[231]

Higher rates of suicide in the biological parents of adoptees who commit suicide than in the adoptive parents are indicative of a significant genetic influence on suicide. A Danish study based on all the adoptions in Copenhagen between 1924 and 1947 looked for genetic and environmental effects by examining the causes of death for the adoptees and their biological relatives. Within this group of adoptees, 57 eventually committed suicide. They were matched with a control group of other adoptees for age, sex, social class, and time spent in institutions or with biological parents. Twelve of the biological relatives of the adoptees who committed suicide had also committed suicide; only two of the biological relatives of the adoptees who had not committed suicide had killed themselves. None of the adopting relatives of either the suicide or control group committed suicide.[231] This was a highly significant difference, suggesting a genetic basis. This finding was replicated in a second study of Danish adoptees in which a much higher rate of suicide was observed among the relatives of the adoptees with mood disorders compared to those with no history of psychiatric illness.[231] This phenomenon of familial clustering of depression is limited to neither a particular time nor a particular place. Myrna Weissman, an epidemiologist at Columbia University, followed the offspring of moderately to severely depressed and nondepressed parents for 20 years to a mean age of 35 years and observed that the risks of anxiety disorders, major depression, and substance abuse dependence occurred among the offspring of the depressed at nearly three times the rate as in the offspring of the nondepressed. The period of highest risk of serious depression occurred between ages 15 years and 25 years and predominantly in females. She concluded, "The offspring of depressed parents constitute a high-risk group for psychiatric and medical problems, which begin early and continue through adulthood."[232] These studies represent an alternative way of thinking about the genesis of mental illness. Parents who are cold, withdrawn, or abusive may be increasing the risk of mental illness in their offspring not only because they are non-nurturing but also because they are transmitting genes that may alter the thoughts and moods of their children.

My friend, Ann Pulver, has made the focus of her career the study of mental illnesses among Ashkenazi Jews— schizophrenia and manic-depressive disease. Ann and I have known each other for a long time, because we sat in adjacent cubicles when we were postdoctoral fellows in medical genetics at Johns Hopkins. From her graduate student days, Ann has studied the causality of mental illnesses, originally from studying features of people hospitalized at mental health facilities in Maryland, later from studying their DNA and the DNA of their family members. During our fellowship days, her work focused on season of birth and mental illness. Ann and her co-investigators observed that schizophrenics were more likely to be born in the winter rather than in another season. This suggested that a seasonal factor, such as viral infection, malnutrition, vitamin deficiency, or obstetrical complication, could damage an infant's brain and predispose the child to psychosis later in life.[233]

More recently, her work has focused on a possible genetic basis for schizophrenia and bipolar disease among Ashkenazi Jews. Like Goodman, she emphatically does not believe that these conditions are more prevalent among Jews. Rather, she argues that because this group has historically married within the group, fewer disease-predisposing genes have entered the gene pool, thereby simplifying the search. Ann has not been alone in her choice of a historically endogamous group for studying the genetic causes of mental illness. Similar approaches have been employed among the Amish, the Finns, Icelandics, and geographically isolated tribes in Central and South America, as well as Pacific Island populations.

For both schizophrenia and bipolar I disease (the form of the disease characterized by disabling bouts of mania and depression), Ann has identified variant genes in the brain-signaling pathway that is mediated by the chemical glutamate.[234] Schizophrenia is characterized by hallucinations, delusions, lack of motivation, and absence of experiencing pleasure. There can be overlap in the presentation of these conditions—a majority of individuals with bipolar I experience hallucinations or delusions. In fact, recognizing the overlap of these conditions, the diagnosis schizoaffective disorder was developed to categorize patients who have both the mood disorder of bipolar disease and the thought disorder of schizophrenia, so it is plausible to anticipate that they might share an underlying biochemical and signaling defect.

Ann's interest in studying schizophrenia among Ashkenazi Jews is shared by Ariel Darvasi, a geneticist at Hebrew University. Originally, Ariel started IDGene Pharmaceuticals, a company whose focus was gene identification for common conditions among Ashkenazi Jews, including juvenile and adult-onset diabetes mellitus, schizophrenia, Parkinson and Alzheimer diseases, asthma, and breast and colon cancer. He has argued, "The use of the Ashkenazi Jewish founder population has several advantages, primarily in reducing genetic variance and avoiding false-positive results due to population stratification."[235] The focus of IDGene was similar to that of deCode Genetics, a company established in Iceland to study common diseases among the highly inter-related Icelandic population. Both efforts were very successful in their identification of genetic variants that increase risk for common diseases; yet neither succeeded as a commercial entity. The considerable patient resources of IDGene have since been transferred to Hebrew University in Jerusalem in the form of the Hebrew University Genetic Resource (HUGR), where it is now available to international investigators for studying the genetic basis of common diseases.

Ariel's team was the first to show association between variants in the *catechol-O-methyltransferase (COMT)* gene and schizophrenia, a gene whose product breaks down a class of neurotransmitters called catecholamines. Both Ann and Ariel have had other significant observations about a genetic basis for mental illnesses, but Ann has not replicated Ariel's finding for *COMT* genetic variation and schizophrenia, perhaps because the diagnoses of her groups are different. In fact, as of now, there is no specific story about how genetic predispositions, exposures prior to birth, and patterns of rearing cause bipolar disease and schizophrenia. It is not even clear that Ann and Ariel's hypotheses about studying Ashkenazi Jews to reduce the complexity for understanding the genetic basis of these conditions is correct. Thus, there is no basis for predicting which groups may be at risk for certain mental illnesses based on their genetic profiles of their patterns of rearing, although one might foresee that happening in the future. In fact, one can foresee a potentially new and unfortunate genetic typology that will lead to a form of stereotyping based on genetics—this group is predisposed to schizophrenia; that group is predisposed to depression—even when fairly small differences are observed between groups. Undoubtedly, this form of genetic stereotyping will be applied to other conditions as well.

One can imagine that future genetic studies might try to identify a common cause for creativity and depression. Jamison has observed that at least 20 studies have found that highly creative individuals are more likely than the general population to suffer from depression and manic-depressive illness. She observed, "Clearly, mood disorders are not required for great accomplishment, and most people who suffer from mood disorders are not particularly accomplished. But the evidence is compelling that the creative are disproportionately affected by these conditions."[231] Yet most of these studies and the resulting catalogs that they produce tend to focus on highly accomplished writers, composers, and visual artists, fueling speculation about the artistic temperament. British psychiatrist Felix Post's investigation of 291 famous scientists, inventors, thinkers, scholars, statesmen, national leaders, painters, sculptors, composers, novelists, and playwrights was based on having adequate biographical materials on these men to develop psychiatric diagnoses based on DSM-III-R criteria, when appropriate.[236] He observed that in each category, 40% or more of the men had "potentially handicapping traits of DSM personality disorders," of which 21% or more had episodic disabling disorders. Notably, among the scientists, the two progenitors of human genetics, Mendel and Galton, were deemed to have "severe" psychopathology, and Galton's cousin, Charles Darwin, was deemed to have "marked" psychopathology. The writers, artists, and composers as a group had a far higher proportion of members with severe psychopathology than the others. These observations were reinforced in a study of fifteen twentieth-century Abstract Expressionist artists of the New York School performed in the mid-1990s by a group of Harvard Medical School psychiatrists. They observed more than 50% of the artists in this group had some form of mental illness, usually mood disorders and preoccupation with death, often compounded by alcohol abuse. At least six sought treatment, three were hospitalized for psychiatric problems, two committed suicide, two died in motor vehicle accidents while driving, and two others had fathers who committed suicide. Seven of 15 artists were dead by age 60 years.[237] Jamison's work on manic-depressive disease and creativity (discussed in her book, *Touched with Fire*) focused on visual and literary artists.[238] The pedigrees that she presented for these writers and artists demonstrated many family members affected with depression. Extrapolating from her findings, Jamison proposed a genetic link between depression and particular forms of visual and auditory creativity.

So the pendulum has swung toward nature in the nature–nurture debate originated by Galton. The role of genes in determining whether we are pious or wayward, intellectual or a slacker, generous or miserly is likely to be investigated in coming decades. Twin studies have pointed the way toward examining whether these traits have high heritabilities. Association studies will follow to identify the genetic variants that predispose to specific behavioral types, and both civil law and religious law will be challenged to account for whether an individual predisposed to dysphoric impulses has the free will to contain them. The observation that virtually no trait is completely genetically determined and that environmental modifiers have a role for all traits will provide a conceptual underpinning for civil and religious authorities that individuals must engage in the struggle for restraining their dysphoric impulses. Specific therapies, both medical and psychological, will continue to have a role in helping individuals to control their impulses, and genetic testing will likely have a role in defining who will respond to specific therapies and what the nature of that response might be.

Genetic research is not all about moral dilemma related to great discovery. It has been benefited people in many ways. Within my field of medical genetics, genetic knowledge has reduced suffering and improved peoples' lives. Three examples stand out. Since the early 1970s, screening for Tay-Sachs disease has been available for Ashkenazi Jews.[72] This has taken many forms, both community-based and medically based. Thousands of people come each year for genetic testing. Sometimes it is a couple who is already in a pregnancy and is trying to decide whether they should have prenatal diagnosis via amniocentesis. Sometimes it is a couple who had a child with a fatal disease, such as Tay-Sachs, and is trying to decide whether they should have an embryo biopsy and in vitro fertilization with only normal embryos. Sometimes it is a young couple at Yeshiva University that is contemplating marriage but wants to know the genetic information before they become serious. More than a million people have been tested for Tay-Sachs carrier status. The number of births of children with Tay-Sachs disease number only 4 or 5 per year where they used to be 40 to 50 per year prior

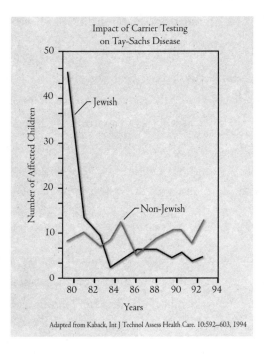

Figure 5.3. Effect of genetic carrier screening on reducing the incidence of Tay-Sachs disease. With screening, Tay-Sachs went from being a Jewish-predominant to a non-Jewish-predominant disease. (See color figure.)

to genetic screening (Figure 5.3). Currently, Ashkenazi Jews are screened for 17 conditions. In the future, it is likely to be more as the genetic basis for more conditions is identified. New genetic testing programs are being developed for Sephardic and Middle Eastern Jews, because having a child with a fatal genetic disease is a tragedy. In the past, when a couple had a child with a genetic disease, often they stopped having children. But today screening for genetic diseases has been accepted into the mainstream of Judaism.

In his book on bioethics, Rabbi Elliot Dorf wrote:

> For some time young Ashkenazic Jews have been warned to be tested for Tay-Sachs disease...A few rabbis in the Orthodox community object to testing for fear that discovery of defective genes in the fetus will lead to abortion...Carriers should, however, try to marry people who are not themselves carriers so as to avoid the possibility of producing a child with the disease...According to the vast majority of rabbis of all streams of Judaism, however, an abortion of a fetus afflicted with Tay-Sachs disease would be warranted. If both members of the couples are carriers for a particular disease, they may use donor semen or eggs as a way of avoiding the possibility that they will conceive a child who suffers from the disease...They may also use birth control and adopt children.[239]

A second way in which genetic knowledge has reduced suffering has been in the treatment of genetic disease. One of the dramatic examples is the treatment of Gaucher disease, a disease

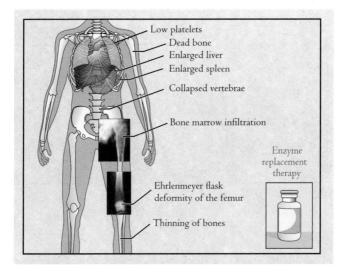

Figure 5.4. Effects of treating Gaucher disease with enzyme-replacement
therapy with alleviation of many of the pathological features. (See color figure.)

that is similar to Tay-Sachs, because it results in accumulation
of fatty material in the lysosomes of cells—both are *lysosomal
storage diseases* (Figure 5.4).[240] Usually, Gaucher does not affect
the nervous system, and usually it is not fatal but may be as the
result of uncontrolled bleeding. People with Gaucher disease
can be quite disabled with bone pain, hip fractures, and large
spleens. But knowledge of the genetic defect in Gaucher disease
has led to a specific therapy in which the enzyme that is missing from the people who have the disease is replaced by injec-
tion. The results of treatment are dramatic—normal bleeding
times, reduced bone pain, elimination of hip fractures. Gaucher
was the first disease in which enzyme-replacement therapy was

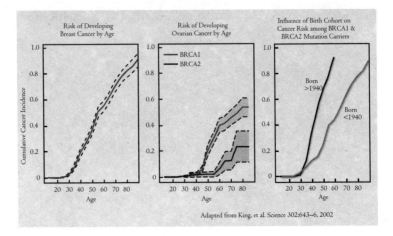

Adapted from King, et al. Science 302:643–6, 2002

Figure 5.5. Significant discoveries from studying *BRCA1/2* mutations in
Ashkenazi Jewish populations—(Left) similar risk of developing breast cancer by
age 80 years, regardless of whether a woman is a *BRCA1* or *BRCA2* mutation
carrier; (Center) Higher risk of developing ovarian cancer by age 80 years, if a
woman is a *BRCA1* rather than *BRCA2* mutation carrier; (Right) Apparent earlier
onset of breast cancer if a woman was born after 1940. (See color figure.)

used successfully. Now another form of treatment is underway
that prevents the accumulation of the fatty substance from the
start.

A third success story is genetic testing for breast and ovarian cancer (Figure 5.5).[241] Often cancer runs in families and
women with mothers, sisters, aunts, and cousins with breast and
ovarian cancer come from high-risk families. Rosalind Franklin,
a young English Orthodox Jewish woman, came from such a
family.[242] Along with James Watson and Francis Crick, she discovered the structure of DNA. She died of ovarian cancer at the

age of 37 years. It was by studying just such families with early-onset breast and ovarian cancer, such as Rosalind Franklin's, that the genes now known as *BRCA1* and *BRCA2* were identified. Among Ashkenazi Jews, three mutations are common and make genetic testing simple and relatively inexpensive. A common *BRCA1* mutation has also been found among Iranian Jews. And here, too, genetic testing has led to prevention of cancers with preservation of life.

Ashkenazi Jews may also be in the vanguard for population-based genetic screening for breast and ovarian cancer risk. In 2009, Rubinstein and her colleagues from Northwestern University Medical School and North Shore University Health System published an article, "A call for dialogue."[243] Her premise was that almost half of Ashkenazi Jewish individuals identified with *BRCA1/2* mutations have a negative family history for cancer and that this confounds efforts toward presymptomatic carrier identification. Their model predicted that a genetic screening program would result in 2,811 fewer cases of ovarian cancer, with a life expectancy gain of 1.83 quality-adjusted life years among carriers. At a cost of $460 for founder mutation testing, the cost of the program would be $8,300 (discounted) per year of quality-adjusted life gained. Their recommendations were at odds with earlier recommendations of the U.S. Preventive Services Task Force that population-based genetic screening for *BRCA1/2* should not be offered.

Rubinstein's recommendation was based in part on an as-yet unpublished study by Levy-Lahad from Shaare Zedek

Medical Centre in Jerusalem.[244] Levy-Lahad recruited more than 7,200 men and identified more than 150 families with *BRCA1/2* mutations. They counseled and tested women in these families, many of whom were not aware that they were at increased risk and were not undergoing screening. Their results suggested that cancer risks for carriers are just as high in these families as in carriers from high-risk families. The website for the Breast Cancer Research Foundation noted, "The researchers are continuing their study, and if more robust risk estimates remain high, they may determine it is justified to offer BRCA1/BRCA2 screening in the general population."[245] Similar studies have been underway at Women's College Hospital in Toronto and University College London. Some have called this "No-brainer testing."

But is that true? Genetic testing without adequate genetic counseling can lead to fear and anxiety. Myriad Genetics conducted such a television marketing campaign in 2002. On the Genome.gov website, under "Direct to Consumer Marketing of Genetic Tests," it was noted:

> In Denver, one of the cities in which the ads ran, cancer genetics centers noted a 300 percent increase in calls from women interested in BRACAnalysis, but a 30 percent decrease in referral of high risk women during the campaign. These data signal a potential failure of the ads to reach the target population of women most likely to benefit from the information gained from BRACAnalysis. Further research

showed that the advertisements did not accurately portray the test's ability to predict cancer or encourage consumers to contact their health care provider.[246]

The availability of such a program can create an elite status for Ashkenazi Jews but not for other Jewish or non-Jewish groups, where comparable tests are not available. As Rubinstein suggested, this is the time for a dialogue.

Such a dialogue will touch on the fact that contemporary Jews are making spousal choices and using genetic information for disease treatment, disease prevention, and embryo selection to determine who future Jews will be. Many Jews are marrying outside their traditional communities yet raising their offspring within those communities. People who might have died from cancer at a young age are identified and their diseases are being prevented, enabling them to transmit genes that might otherwise have been lost. Young men and women who are both carriers for Tay-Sachs disease are deciding not to marry. In the process, they do not have children with Tay-Sachs disease, but the frequency of the Tay-Sachs disease mutations increases within the population. So through their behavior and medical treatments, contemporary Jewry is transforming the genetic makeup of future Jewry.

SIX

—

IDENTITY

Albert Einstein arguably may have been the most famous Jew of the twentieth century (Figure 6.1). As his biographer Walter Isaacson noted, "When he arrived in New York in April, [1921], he was greeted by adoring throngs as the world's first scientific celebrity, one who also happened to be a gentle icon of humanist values and a living patron saint for Jews."[247] Yet over the course of his lifetime, he became a committed Jew and Zionist and, eventually, was offered the presidency of Israel, an honor that he declined. Near the end of his life in 1955 he stated, "My relationship to the Jewish people has become my strongest human tie."[248] Einstein explained the route to his Jewishness in his popular 1934 book, *The World As I See It:* "The pursuit of knowledge for its own sake, an almost fanatical love

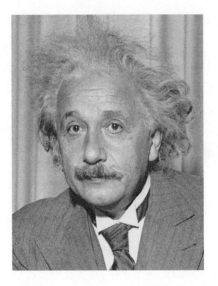

Figure 6.1. Photo of Albert Einstein, Swiss, German, and American physicist, famous for his theories of relativity that transformed physics. In 1955, he stated, "My relationship to the Jewish people has become my strongest human tie."

of justice, and the desire for personal independence—these are the features of the Jewish tradition which make me thank my stars that I belong to it." He went on to note:

> In the philosophical sense there is, in my opinion, no specific Jewish outlook. Judaism seems to me to be concerned almost exclusively with the moral attitude in life and to life. I look upon it as the essence of an attitude to life which is incarnate in the Jewish people rather than the essence of laws laid down in the Torah and interpreted in the Talmud.[249]

Einstein was emphatic that his Jewish identity was not religiously motivated. "In your letter," he told the rabbis of Berlin in 1921, who had urged him to become a dues-paying member of the Jewish religious community, "I notice that the word Jew is ambiguous in that it refers (1) to nationality and origin, (2) to the faith. I am a Jew in the first sense, not the second."[250]

So Einstein highlighted several of the features that foster Jewish identity—nationality (or race or group membership), the culture emanating from group membership, and shared religious belief. In the United States, religion remains a powerful force in Jewish identity, as do an inner commitment to being Jewish and significant Jewish friendship ties. The *National Jewish Population Survey of 2000–2001* observed, "Most American Jewish adults observe in some way the High Holidays, Passover and Chanukah. Majorities also read a Jewish newspaper or magazine or books with Jewish content, regard being Jewish as very important, and report that half or more of their close friends are Jewish."[37] This survey is sponsored every 10 years by the philanthropic United Jewish Communities and Jewish Federations of North America to understand the size of the North American Jewish population and its key characteristics. The survey found that one-fourth to a one-third of the population is very religiously and communally inclined. This inclination is manifested by lighting Sabbath candles, keeping a kosher home, attending religious services at least monthly, belonging to a Jewish Community Center or other Jewish

organization, making financial contributions to Jewish charities, volunteering in Jewish social service agencies, participating in Jewish adult education programs, and visiting Israel
twice or more. One-third to one-half of the population is
moderately engaged in a variety of Jewish behaviors, including
belonging to a synagogue as an individual or as a household,
making a personal or household donation to a Jewish cause
outside the Federation system, using the Internet for Jewish
purposes, and participating in cultural activities with Jewish
content. Zionism is a feature of this American view of Jewish
identity. Beyond religious and cultural observance and philan-
thropy, the number of visits to Israel tends to correlate with
an individual's Jewish engagement.

In his book, *The Holocaust in American Life*, Peter Novick
observed these statistics, but did not view them to be sufficiently compelling to provide the basis for a distinctive Jewish
identity in the United States.[251] He wrote:

> These days American Jews can't define their Jewishness on
> the basis of distinctively Jewish religious beliefs, since most
> don't have much in the way of distinctively Jewish beliefs.
> They can't define it by distinctively Jewish cultural traits,
> since most don't have any of these either. American Jews
> are sometimes said to be united by their Zionism, but if so,
> it is of a thin and abstract variety; most have never visited
> Israel; most contribute little to, and know even less about,
> that country.

Rather, he has observed that the Holocaust (the extermination of 6 million Jews by the Nazis and their sympathizers) is a major unifying force. In his words,

> What American Jews *do* have in common is the knowledge that but for their parents' or (more often) grandparents' or great-grandparents' immigration, they would have shared the fate of European Jewry. Within an increasingly diverse and divided American Jewry, this became the historical foundation of the endlessly repeated but empirically dubious slogan, "We are one."

Novick went on to say, "Many Jewish commentators have warned that a Holocaust-centered Judaism would not work to ensure Jewish survival—that it would be a turn-off, alienating the young." In practice, it has not worked that way because American culture has embraced the Holocaust as a universal example of evil in the world. As a result, over the past 40 years, the Holocaust has come to represent an American memory, not just a Jewish memory. The Holocaust is, as Novick has noted, an "antidote for innocence." Teaching of the Holocaust in public schools has been legislatively mandated in a number of states— the 1994 New York law cited the following:

> The legislature finds, recognizes and affirms the importance to pupils of learning to appreciate the sanctity of life and the dignity of the individual. Pupils must develop the following, "a respect for each person as a unique individual, and understand

the importance of a universal concern for ethics and human rights." Therefore, the legislature recognizes the importance of teaching our youth ethical and moral behavior specifically relating to human rights violations, genocide issues, and slavery, as well as the Holocaust.[252]

The Mississippi statute went on to amplify this point by noting, "All people should remember the horrible atrocities committed at that time and other times in human history as the result of bigotry and tyranny, and therefore should continually rededicate themselves to the principles of human rights and equal protection under the laws of a democratic society."[253] On a national level, the U. S. Congress created the U. S. Holocaust Memorial Museum as a permanent living memorial and established annual Days of Remembrance to commemorate the victims of the Holocaust.[254] Since 1982, members of the museum staff have organized and led the national Days of Remembrance ceremony in the U.S. Capitol Rotunda. This ceremony includes participation by members of Congress and the White House staff, members of the diplomatic corps, Holocaust survivors, World War II liberators, and community leaders. Thus, in a curious turn of events, remembrance of the Holocaust has become a pro-Semitic, rather than an anti-Semitic, experience. It is also a safeguard against the kind of assimilation of Einstein's European contemporaries, who often felt more German or French than Jewish, only to discover that their European neighbors did not share their views. Helene Berr, a young French woman who died in the Holocaust, kept a diary that survived. Her journal entry on December 31, 1943, typified the assimilation that she experienced:

> When I write the word *Jew*, I am not saying exactly what I mean, because for me that distinction does not exist: I do not feel different from other people, I will never think of myself as a member of a separate human group, and perhaps that is why I suffer so much, because I don't understand it at all.[255]

During Einstein's era, anti-Semitism was common in the United States and had its own cohesive force among Jews. Jews were excluded from universities, clubs, and professions. Sometimes this anti-Semitism was the official policy of the U.S. government, as typified by the refusal to accept larger numbers of European Jewish immigrants at the Evian conference on Jewish immigration from Nazi-occupied countries in 1938 or by the refusal to bomb the rail lines to Auschwitz in 1945 to prevent Jews from being transported to the death camp.[256] Sometimes this anti-Semitism was part of everyday social contact, such as that described in the popular novel and subsequent movie *Gentleman's Agreement*.[257] In this story, the widowed, gentile journalist, Philip Schuyler Green, adopted a Jewish identity as "Phil Green" to write about first-hand experiences with anti-Semitism. The bigotry that he experienced was sometimes subtle, other times more overt. Both Phil and his son, Tommy, readily encountered anti-Semitic remarks, with Tommy being called a "dirty Jew" by his schoolmates. The anti-Semitism of Phil's fiancée, Kathy Lacey, and her social set in Darien, Connecticut, was the major source of conflict in the book—such as the decision of some of Kathy's friends to boycott the party celebrating her engagement to a "Jew." Even Phil's secretary, Elaine Wales (née Estelle Wilovsky), concealed her Jewish identity and practiced her own brand of anti-Semitism, worrying that an open hiring policy would attract the "wrong Jews" and ruin things for the few Jews who worked at their magazine. This pervasive anti-Semitism in everyday life was not merely the stuff of fiction. In *Outliers*, Gladwell described how some of the Jewish superlawyers of today were not hired by white-shoe law firms in the 1950s, because they were not "like us."[258] The direct personal experience of anti-Semitism and the recall of stories, such as Phil Green's, created a bonding among Jews in the United States in the mid-twentieth century and even earlier.

The 2000–2001 *National Jewish Population Survey* has shown that anti-Semitism is simply not present at levels where it would serve as a threat and cohesive force. The writers of the *American Jewish Yearbook 2007* noted:

> The American Jewish community in the U.S.—the largest concentration of Jews in the world outside Israel—experienced remarkably low levels of expression of anti-Semitic expression, both behavioral and attitudinal in 2006. This followed a 50-year pattern that reflected the strengths of a pluralistic society, even as intergroup tensions in general continued to concern political leaders and social analysts.[259]

This has translated into a different set of feelings about being Jewish in the United States, with most contemporary American Jews viewing themselves as Einstein did—both assimilated and Jewish.

In 1984, Silberman documented this transition from an anti-Semitic age in his influential book, *A Certain People: American Jews and Their Lives Today*.[260] This book provided a sunny view of his fellow Jews in the latter part of the twentieth century. His message was reassuring that American Jews had successfully weathered both anti-Semitism and assimilation and retained their Jewishness. Through research and anecdote, Silberman described how Jews achieved that comfortable state in America. Silberman explained, "In the past, Jews remained Jews for one of three reasons: because they believed that was what God demanded of them; because they were born into an organic community with powerful sanctions and rewards; or because anti-Semites would not permit them to become anything else." In *A Certain People*, Silberman discarded religion and anti-Semitism as reasons for retaining Jewish identity in favor of community. He claimed, "None of these factors can be relied upon today. Although American Jews are keenly aware of anti-Semitism, there is no longer enough of it to hold the community together." In the process, he was claiming for American Jews the transition of a community that has reached its third generation since the time of immigration and the pride that had come from "making it" within American society as a member of a small ethnic minority. Silberman, a former editor at *Fortune* magazine, was a writer of some clout, having previously published several successful books that provided critiques of race (*Crisis in Black and White*), education (*Crisis in the Classroom: The Remaking of American Education*), and criminality (*Criminal Violence, Criminal Justice: Criminals, Police, Courts and Prisons in America*). His book, *Crisis in the Classroom*, was widely cited in public debates about educational reform during the 1970s.

Yet, the transition that Silberman described was not complete. He wrote, "It is not surprising, therefore, that most American Jews continue to feel more comfortable in the company of other Jews." In one recent survey, for example, 61 percent of the respondents reported that all, almost all, or most of their friends were Jewish. These feelings were not unique to Jews. Regardless of their success, older Italian-Americans like older Jews, found it hard to lose the sense that they were "guests" in someone else's country. Younger Italian-Americans, like younger Jews, did not bear that burden of self-consciousness and perceived themselves as full-fledged Americans and free to take pride in their ethnic identity.[260]

Not all members of the Jewish community embraced Silberman's triumphalism. In his review, Hertzberg worried that crises still fueled the basis for Jewish identity. He feared an eventual full-blown peace in the Middle East would eliminate one of the few remaining crises that galvanized Jews' attention—in his words, "successive generations of the Jewish bourgeoisie will not find other causes to engage their attention."[261] He worried also that the pull toward assimilation with intermarriage rates hovering at 50% would outweigh the religious and cultural revival described in *A Certain People*. Criticizing Silberman, he stated, "He simply rejects out of hand the possibility that this unique hospitality makes relatively painless assimilation, an even easier choice for many Jews than the choice to engage in separatist activism within the Jewish community." Another contemporary Silberman critic, Walter Goodman, took a more balanced view by pointing out, "Assimilation can mean a more secure identity or the loss of identity."[262] Yet, over the past generation, the loss of identity simply predicted by Hertzberg and Goodman has not materialized for contemporary American Jews as it did for Helen Berr and her contemporaries.

The experiences of Jews in America and other Western countries where they have assimilated in national life with the attendant loss of anti-Semitism differs in some ways from those in countries where Jews have been viewed as a people apart from the dominant population, and from Israel, where Jews constitute the dominant population. Based on her own life experience, journalist Masha Gessen has claimed that American Jews are the only people in the world who believe that Jews are not a race. She has stated, "It's lovely to think that being Jewish is a religious tradition, but you sort of have to have the luxury of the United States of America to be able to do that. Elsewhere, it is actually whom you're born to."[263] Gessen was listed as Jewish on her birth certificate, because she was born in the Soviet Union to people who themselves were listed as Jewish on their birth certificates, not because they were religiously observant. In fact, in the Soviet Union, *Jewish* was 1 of 69 distinct nationalities. In the beginning of the 1990s, this nationality field was removed from Russian passports.[264]

In Israel, being Jewish or Arab (rather than Israeli) is also a nationality—Israeli is a citizenship. This decision originated with the founders of Israel, who stated in Israel's Declaration of Independence that Israel would be a Jewish, rather than a secular, state.[265] The Law of Return (1950) provided the legal basis by declaring that Jewish people everywhere have the right to come to Israel.[266] This included Jews by choice who converted to Judaism through the Orthodox, Reform, or Conservative denominations. The religious parties in the Knesset sought to define conversion as having been supervised by the Orthodox rabbinate. This created tension with American Jewish leaders, who insisted that Israel could not delegitimize Reform and Conservative conversions. Bowing to Israeli religious politics, the Knesset decided that conversions must have been religious and not secular and, if Reform and Conservative, must have occurred abroad, as only Orthodox conversions are recognized within Israel. The Jewish Ancestry Amendment of 1970 extended the right of return to the child and grandchild of a Jew, the spouse of a Jew, the spouse of a child of a Jew, and the spouse of a grandchild of a Jew.[266] The inclusive scope of this amendment provides sanctuary in Israel to anyone who would have been persecuted under the Nazi Nuremberg Laws of 1935.[267] Under the Law of Return, a Jew can be excluded from Israeli citizenship if he or she "is engaged in an activity directed against the Jewish people; or is likely to endanger public health or the security of the State."[265] Jews who have committed serious crimes or who are fugitives in other countries (unless persecution victims) can be denied the right of return. The law also excludes any people who were Jewish but voluntarily changed their religion. In 1989, the Supreme Court of Israel decided that Messianic Judaism that combines elements of Judaism and Christianity is not the Jewish religion, so that people who have become Messianic Jews are also excluded.[268] The Law of Return does not determine Israeli citizenship; it merely allows for Jews and their eligible descendants to permanently relocate within Israel.

The Nationality Law (1952) governs how individuals can gain Israeli citizenship.[266] By passing this law, Israeli Parliament (Knesset) made a clear distinction from the right to immigrate to Israel that was provided by the Law of Return and the right to citizenship. The Nationality Law stated that citizenship is granted to people who were born in Israel to a mother or a father who is an Israeli citizen; to people who are born outside Israel, if their father or mother holds Israeli citizenship; to people who are born after the death of one of their Israeli parents; or to people who were born in Israel and who have never had any nationality if they apply between their 18th and 25th birthdays and have been residents of Israel for 5 consecutive years, immediately preceding the day of the filing of their application. The net effect of these laws has been to increase immigration levels by expanding the base of eligible people. In the process of allowing more secular Jews and their non-Jewish spouses to immigrate, the then secular leadership of Israel sought on the one hand to encourage immigration of people sympathetic to the view of Israel as a Jewish state and on the other hand to minimize and undermine the influence of the religious parties in Israeli politics and society. In his book, *The Invention of the Jewish People*, Sand points out that the concept of a Jewish nation and nationhood (derived from the verb *nascere* or "to beget") is a means for establishing political and cultural coherence.[269] Elaborating further, he stated:

> But the Law of the Return and the associated Law of Citizenship were direct products of an ethnic nationalist worldview, designed to provide a legal concept for the concept that the State of Israel belongs to the Jews of the world. As Ben-Gurion declared at the start of parliamentary debate on the Law of the Return, "This is not a Jewish state only because most of its inhabitants are Jews. It is a state for the Jews wherever they may be, and for any Jews who wish to be here."

Yet, one does not have to be Jewish to benefit from living in Israel. Israel's Declaration of Independence called for equality of social and political rights, regardless of religion, race, or sex. Israeli citizens and permanent residents are guaranteed rights by a set of basic laws. The Israeli Supreme Court has interpreted *Basic Law: Human Dignity and Liberty* and *Basic Law: Freedom of Occupation* as guaranteeing equal rights for all Israeli citizens, although some differences exist. Military service is mandatory

Box 6.I. Law of Return 5710–1950, enabling Diaspora Jews to immigrate to Israel.

Law of Return 5710–1950

RIGHT OF ALIYAH

I. Every Jew has the right to come to this country as an oleh*

OLEH'S VISA

2. (a) Aliyah shall be by oleh's visa.

   (b) An oleh's visa shall be granted to every Jew who has expressed his desire to settle in Israel, unless the Minister of Immigration is satisfied that the applicant

     (I) is engaged in an activity directed against the Jewish people; or

     (2) is likely to endanger public health or the security of the State.

OLEH'S CERTIFICATE

3. (a) A Jew who has come to Israel and subsequent to his arrival has expressed his desire to settle in Israel may, while still in Israel, receive an oleh's certificate.

   (b) The restrictions specified in section 2(b) shall apply also to the grant of an oleh's certificate,

(*continued*)

Box 6.1. (Continued)

but a person shall not be regarded as endangering public health on account of an illness contracted after his arrival in Israel.

RESIDENTS AND PERSONS BORN IN THIS COUNTRY

4. Every Jew who has immigrated into this country before the coming into force of this Law, and every Jew who was born in this country, whether before or after the coming into force of this Law, shall be deemed to be a person who has come to this country as an oleh under this Law.

IMPLEMENTATION AND REGULATIONS

5. The Minister of Immigration is charged with the implementation of this Law and may make regulations as to any matter relating to such implementation and also as to the grant of oleh's visas and oleh's certificates to minors up to the age of 18 years.

DAVID BEN-GURION
Prime Minister

MOSHE SHAPIRA
Minister of Immigration

YOSEF SPRINZAK

Acting President of the State
Chairman of the Knesset

*Translator's Note: Aliyah means immigration of Jews

for virtually all citizens and permanent, although exemptions
are granted to the ultra-Orthodox and Arab Israelis. Marriage
is regulated by religious, rather than civil, authorities. Marriage
among Jews is regulated by the Israeli (Orthodox) rabbinate.

Writing in *Commentary* magazine, journalist Hillel Halkin
has described how in Israel, Jewishness is now a secular, legal
category as well as a religious category and that both categories are linked because marriage and conversion are controlled by the Orthodox rabbinate.[270] He has noted, "Yet
the more contentious the question of who is a Jew becomes,
the more this law divides Jews rather than unites them." He
has explained the dilemma of hundreds of thousands of
immigrants mostly from the former Soviet Union who were
able to enter Israel under the Law of the Return because
they were either married to Jews or had a Jewish father or
grandfather. This period of mass migration of Soviet Jews
created mistrust between secular and religious Jews. Most
Soviet Jews and their children cannot have a wedding in
Israel, because they are not recognized as Jews and because

civil marriage does not exist. Although many would like to
be recognized as Jews and might even be willing to undergo
a religious conversion, they have been deterred because the
rabbinate has required potential converts to promise living
an Orthodox life. Halkin has gone on to describe how a conversion was annulled retroactively by the rabbinate, because
such a promise was not kept. The rabbinate has argued that it
has been forced to require more rigorous standards, because
Israeli society has become very secular. This has precluded
the "honor system" for determining Jewish identity that
operated in Israel in the past.

Halkin has also noted, "Even Israelis whose Jewishness
might appear to be beyond question now find themselves
questioned about it." A case in point was his Israeli-born
daughter, who is listed as "Jewish" on her Israeli ID card. To
obtain a marriage license, she was required to provide proof
of her Jewishness in the form a letter from an Orthodox
rabbi in the United States attesting to the Orthodox nature
of the parents' wedding ceremony in New York. Had her parents been married in Israel, their Jewishness would have been
rabbinically certified and that would have been considered
proof of the daughter's Jewishness. Had they been married
in a non-Orthodox ceremony in the United States, their non-
Orthodox rabbi might not be trusted to have vetted them
properly.

Gorenberg has written, "More than any other issue, the
question of 'Who is a Jew?' has repeatedly roiled relations

between Israel and American Jewry. Psychologically, it is an argument over who belongs to the family."²⁷¹ Halkin has amplified this point:

> For such secular Israelis, the idea of biological Jewishness is an embarrassing anachronism. Secular Zionism, after all, set out to normalize Jewish existence. Surely, they reason, its goal should therefore be to make Israelis a people whose identity is based, like that of other peoples, on territory, language, and culture rather than on shared blood ties.²⁷⁰

But the issue of who belongs in the family is not limited to relations between Israel and American Jewry.

The high rate of intermarriage without spousal conversion has led to a backlash within the Jewish community about who belongs in the family. Legal scholar Noah Feldman described having his photographic image removed from the publications of Maimonides, the modern Orthodox day school that he attended as a child growing up in Brookline, Massachusetts. Feldman, a law professor at Harvard University and adjunct senior fellow at the Council on Foreign Relations, recounted an unusual event that followed his 10-year school reunion. He participated in the reunion with his Korean-American girlfriend (who is now his wife). The group photo from the event was touched up so that their images were removed— Photoshopped® out. He wrote in the *New York Sunday Times Magazine*, "Her presence implied the prospect of something that from the standpoint of Orthodox Jewish law could not be recognized: marriage to someone who was not Jewish. That hint was reason enough to keep us out."[272] A very painful experience for Feldman, he went on to note:

> It would be more dramatic if I had been excommunicated like Baruch Spinoza, in a ceremony complete with black candles and a ban on all social contact, a rite whose solemnity reflected the seriousness of its consequences. But in the modern world, the formal communal ban is an anachronism…What remains of the old technique of excommunication is simply non-recognition in the school's formal publications, where my classmates' growing families and considerable accomplishments are joyfully celebrated.

Feldman and his family are not alone. Even with conversion, there has been backlash within the modern Orthodox Jewish community about the Jewishness of a converted spouse and her offspring. Brandeis University professor Jonathan Sarna has written that the number of people in America recognized only by some movements as Jewish may be in the hundreds of thousands—Sarna's figure includes the children of Jewish fathers and non-Jewish mothers.[273] This disagreement has spilled over to Western Europe. In 2007, tension erupted at the London Jewish Free School, a religious day school, when a child was refused admission.[274] He was deemed non-Jewish based on the fact that his mother had converted to Judaism under the aegis of a non-Orthodox religious court (*beit din*). He was actually the third child of a converted Jewish mother to be denied admission to the Jewish Free School within the span of a few years. Outraged, his Jewish-by-birth father sued. The local court ruled in the school's favor, but the appeals court, headed by a Jewish judge, decided that admission on the basis of Jewish birth, rather than Jewish belief, amounted to ethnic, or racial, discrimination! As a result, he ruled that under English law, the determinant for admission should be the child's Jewish beliefs and practices, rather than his lineage.

This belief that Jews constitute a religious, rather than ethnic or racial, group is widespread in the United States and other Western countries. In the United States, the 1997 White House Office of Management and Budget's *Revisions to the Standards for the Classification of Federal Data on Race and Ethnicity* that served as the basis for the 2010 U.S. Census lists *White* as a race for people having European, Middle Eastern, or North African ancestry but does not include *Jewish* as a category.[275] Indeed, *Jewish* has never been a category in the U.S. Census. Yet the genetic studies would seem to refute this.

The evidence for biological Jewishness has become incontrovertible. The answer to Jacobs' 1899 question, "Are Jews Jews?" would seem to be an emphatic yes.[276] As noted earlier, a study by Goldstein and his coworkers demonstrated that it was possible to predict full Ashkenazi Jewish ancestry accurately and with a somewhat lesser degree of certainty for people with one, two, or three Jewish grandparents.[190] The Jewish HapMap Project has extended these findings to people who come from virtually all other Jewish groups, each group representing a genetic cluster that can be defined as a predominant pattern of inheritance that includes a large number of genetic markers.[1] The findings are based on the fact that segments of the genome tend to be shared at a higher frequency among members of a particular Jewish group and at a lesser frequency among members of different Jewish groups. This degree of shared genetic segments is greater among Jews than between Jews and non-Jews. So Jewishness at a genetic level can be characterized as a tapestry with the threads represented as shared segments of DNA and no single thread required for composition of the tapestry. The genetic affiliation of any individual might be higher for a specific Jewish group, rather than for the Jewish people as a whole. There are gaps in this view because the genetics of Jews has not been formally compared to the genetics of all of their historical neighbors. With more research, it might be discerned that genetic exchanges between specific Jewish and non-Jewish groups may have been very high—so that contemporary non-Jews might be identified as having major Jewish ancestry. Thus, there is no rigorous genetic test for Jewishness, nor would the geneticists who have conducted studies in recent generations propose that one should be created. Moreover, such a test would not replace the religious definition of who is a Jew.

Beyond pointing out a biological basis for Jewishness with attendant predilections to certain diseases or other traits, most contemporary human genetic researchers would not propose to engage in such a tussle. In fact, the *American Society of Human*

Genetics, the leading professional society of human geneticists in the United States, issued an advisory against using genetic tests as a basis for predicting personal ancestry.[277] They have pointed out that commercial ancestry testing lacks precision and accuracy and that the psychosocial, ethical, legal, political, and health-related issues have not yet been worked out. The issue is further complicated by the fact that consumers may have access to the named records of others on the website of the company from which they purchased services to search these records for specific genetic matches. In their quest to build more complete and accurate genealogies, these consumers may be outing others who did not have the full Jewish heritage that they had been led to anticipate or did not have the biological grandfathers that they had known as their grandpa or zayda. In the process, they may also be outing individuals who are carriers of high-risk genetic mutations, such as those in the *BRCA1* and *BRCA2* genes, but did not know of this carrier status previously. The genetic frontier, like so many other frontiers of the past and present, is filled with opportunities and risks—both known and unknown.

Views about a genetic basis for Jewishness have been both triumphalist and cautionary. Goldstein has written, "Our genetic heritage is ours to treasure, to explore and to marvel at."[123] However, Entine has warned, "But DNA is certainly a problematical way to establish identity. Despite the understandable excitement that comes with exploring our genetic attic, there is a clear danger in granting far too much explanatory power to the genes…Only genes confer the mystique of indelibility."[122] Sand has taken an even more negative tone, warning:

> Like the field of physical anthropology in the late nineteenth and early twentieth centuries, which released dubious scientific discoveries to a race hungry public, the science of molecular genetics at the end of the twentieth and the beginning of the twenty first century feeds fragmentary discoveries and half-truths to the identity-seeking media.[269]

Are recent discoveries fragmentary and half-truths? I think not, because the molecular genetic studies of which Sand is critical have set the bar higher for discovery, reporting, and acceptance than the race science of a century ago—less standalone observation with more replication and more rigorous statistical testing.

The stakes in genetic analysis are high. It is more than an issue of who belongs in the family and can partake in Jewish life and Israeli citizenship. It touches on the heart of Zionist claims for a Jewish homeland in Israel. One can imagine future disputes about exactly how large the shared Middle Eastern ancestry of Jewish groups has to be to justify Zionist claims. The stakes extend beyond Jews and Israel. Non-Semitic lines of inheritance may absolve Jews from Christ killing—it really wasn't them and their ancestors; it was someone else. And glorious lineages with genetic lines of descent from a king—even a Messiah—may become even more prized than the purported Cohanim modal haplotype was prized over the last decade.

And yet to look over the genetics of Jewish groups and to see the history of the Diaspora woven in is truly a marvel. Co-religionists all, here is what happened as the Jews migrated to new places and saw their numbers wax and wane, as they gained and lost adherents and thrived or were buffeted in these locales by abundance or famine, infectious disease epidemics, and wars and persecution. The population genetics of the Jews is extraordinary in its own right but also models the population genetics of humanity of a whole. Other peoples have migrated to new locales, retained their beliefs, and maintained the genetic continuity with their ancestors. Their histories are retained in their genomes and have been or will be disclosed as their population genetics is revealed.

Much about Jewish genetics remains unknown yet is likely to be discovered in coming decades as more is learned about origins, susceptibility to diseases, and genetics of beneficial traits. The study of Jewish population genetics is potentially fraught with peril. Genetic skeletons are likely to be found, including those that predispose to dread diseases and sociopathic behaviors, but these are unlikely to be unduly prevalent or unique to Jewish groups. On the one hand, the study of Jewish genetics might be viewed as an elitist effort, promoting a certain genetic view of Jewish superiority. On the other, it might provide fodder for anti-Semitism by providing evidence of a genetic basis for undesirable traits that are present among some Jews. These issues will newly challenge the liberal view that humans are created equal, but with genetic liabilities. For me and other geneticists, who have devoted their careers to bringing genetic testing into the community and promoting fairness in the uses of genetic information, this will represent a special challenge.

Jewish genetics is unlikely to replace the hegemony of Jewish law and Jewish culture, nor should it. But as population genetics gains a foothold in the community, with Jews and non-Jews alike wanting to know about their origins, ancestors, and relatives, it will take its place in the formation of group identity alongside shared spirituality, shared social values, and a shared cultural legacy.

REFERENCES

1. Atzmon, G, Hao, L, Pe'er, I, Velez, C, Pearlman, A, Palamara, PF, et al. Abraham's children in the genome era: major Jewish diaspora populations comprise distinct genetic clusters with shared Middle Eastern Ancestry. Am J Hum Genet 86:850–859, 2010.

2. Wade, N. Studies show Jews' genetic similarity. in *New York Times*, New York, 2010.

3. Balter, M. Who are the Jews? Studies spark identity debate. Science 328:1342, 2010.

4. Behar, DM, Yunusbayev, B, Metspalu, M, Metspalu, E, Rosset, S, Parik, J, et al. The genome-wide structure of the Jewish people. Nature 466:238–242, 2010.

5. Darwin, C. *On the Origin of Species by Means of Natural Selection*, (John Murray, London, 1859).

6. Gould, SJ. *Wonderful life: the Burgess Shale and the nature of history*, 347 p. (W.W. Norton, New York, 1989).

7. Leroi, AM. *Mutants : on the form, varieties and errors of the human body*, xv, 431 p. (HarperCollins, London, 2003).

8. Fishberg, M. *The Jews: A Study of Race and Environment*, (Charles Scribner's Sons, New York, 1911).

9. Fishberg, M. The Jews: A study of race and environment. Pop Science Month 49:Sep 257–267, Jan 33–47, 1906–7.

10. Slonim, Y. One of four million. in *Der Tog*, Day Publishing Company, New York, 1925.

11. Goldstein, EL. Fishberg, Maurice. in *American National Biography*, Vol. 8, 1–2 p. eds. Garranty, J.A. & Carnes, M.C. Oxford University Press, New York, 1999.

12. Obituary. Dr. M. Fishberg, 62, is dead. in *New York Times*, New York, 1934.

13. Fishberg, M. Ethnic factors in immigration—A critical view. 1901. Papers read at the National Conference of Charities and Correction, Philadelphia, May, 1906.

14. Fishberg, M. The relative infrequency of tuberculosis among the Jews. American Med 2:695–699, 1901.

15. Fishberg, M. The comparative pathology of the Jews. New York Med J 73:537–543, 576–582, 1901.

16. Fishberg, M. Materials for the physical anthropology of the Eastern European Jews. Ann NY Acad Science 16:155–296, 1905.

17. Fishberg, M. Anthropology of the Jews: I. The cephalic index. Amer Anthropol 4:684–706, 1902.

18. Fishberg, M. Physical anthropology of the Jews: II. Pigmentation. Amer Anthropol 5:89–106, 1902.

19. Fishberg, M. North African Jews. in *Anthropological Papers: Frans Boas Anniversary Volume* 55–63 G.E. Steinart, New York, 1906.

20. Jacobs, J. Anthropology. in *The Jewish Encyclopedia*, Vol. 1, 619–621 p. ed. Adler, C. Funk and Wagnalls, New York, 1906.

21. Epstein, J. The photos of Frédéric Brenner's "Diaspora." in *The Weekly Standard*, 2003.

22. Jacobs, J. *Jewish Statistics: Social, Vital, Anthropometric*, (D. Nutt, London, 1891).

23. Anon. A study of the Jewish race. in *New York Times*, New York, 1911.

24. Kohn, A. Racial purity of the Jew. in *New York Times*, New York, 1905.

25. Jorde, LB & Wooding, SP. Genetic variation, classification and 'race'. Nat Genet 36:S28–33, 2004.

26. Tishkoff, SA & Kidd, KK. Implications of biogeography of human populations for 'race' and medicine. Nat Genet 36:S21–S27, 2004.

27. Risch, N, Burchard, E, Ziv, E & Tang, H. Categorization of humans in biomedical research: genes, race and disease. Genome Biol 3:1–12, 2002.

28. Shanks, H. *Ancient Israel: A Short History from Abraham to the Roman Destruction of the Temple*, (Prentice Hall Biblical Archeological Society, Engelwood Cliffs, NJ, Washington, D.C., 1988).

29. Cohen, SJD. *The Beginnings of Jewishness*, (University of California Press, Berkeley, 1999).

30. House of David Inscription. Biblical Archeolog Rev: 26:74–96, 1994.

31. Ben-Sasson, HH. *A History of the Jewish People*, (Harvard University Press, Cambridge, 1976).

32. Stillman, N. *The Jews of Arab Lands*, (The Jewish Publication Society, Philadelphia, 1991).

33. Weinryb, B. *A History of the Jews in Poland*, (Jewish Publication Society of America, Philadelphia, 1973).

34. Chouraqui, A. *Between East and West; a history of the Jews of North Africa*, xxii, 376 p. (Jewish Publication Society of America, Philadelphia, 1968).

35. Gottheil, R & Reinach, T. Diaspora. In *Jewish Encyclopedia*, Vol. 4, 559–574 p. ed. Adler, C. Funk and Wagnalls, New York, 1906.

36. Koestler, A. *The Thirteenth Tribe*, (Random House, New York, 1976).

37. Berman, ML & Kaplan, EH. *The National Jewish Population Survey 2000–01*, (United Jewish Charities, New York, 2001).

38. Jacobs, J. Statistics. In *Jewish Encyclopedia*, Vol 11, 528–536 p. ed. Adler, C. Funk and Wagnalls, New York, 1906.

39. Goldschmidt, E, ed. *The Genetics of Isolate and Migrant Populations*, Williams and Wilkins, New York, 1963.

40. Sheba, C. Jewish migration in its historical perspective. Isr J Med Sci 7:1333–1341, 1971.

41. Baccelli, G, Durante, F & Ascoli, V. Il Favismo. Il Policlinico Sezione Pratica 22:1505–1536, 1915.

42. Sansone, G, Piga, AM & Segni, G. *Il Favismo*, (Edizioni Minerva Medica, Roma, 1954).

43. Lederer, R. A new form of acute hemolytic anemia. Transact Royal Soc Tropical Med Hygiene 34:387–394, 1940.

44. Alving, AS, Carson, PE, Flanagan, CL & Ickes, CE. Enzymatic deficiency in primaquine-sensitive erythrocytes. Science 124:484–485, 1956.

45. Beutler, E. The hemolytic effect of primaquine and related compounds: a review. Blood 14:103–139, 1959.

46. Motulsky, AG. Drug reactions enzymes, and biochemical genetics. J Am Med Assoc 165:835–837, 1957.

47. Arese, P, Bosia, A, Naitana, A, Gaetani, S, D'Aquino, M & Gaetani, GF. Effect of divicine and isouramil on red cell metabolism in normal and G6PD-deficient (Mediterranean variant)

subjects. Possible role in the genesis of favism. Prog Clin Biol Res 55:725–746, 1981.

47a. Gross RT, Hurwitz RE, Marks PA. Hereditary enzymatic defect in erythrocyte metabolism. J Clin Invest 37:1176–1189, 1958.

48. Adam, A, Sheba, C, Sanger, R, Race, RR, Tippett, P, Hamper, J, et al. Data for X-mapping calculations, Israeli families tested for Xg, G-6-PD and for colour vision. Ann Hum Genet 26:187–194, 1963.

49. Bateson, W. *Mendel's Principles of Heredity: a Defence*, (Cambridge University Press, 1902).

50. Lyon, MF. Gene action in the X-chromosome of the mouse (Mus musculus). Nature 190:372–373, 1961.

51. Beutler, E, Yeh, M & Fairbanks, VF. The normal human female as a mosaic of X-chromosome activity: studies using the gene for G-6-PD-deficiency as a marker. Proc Natl Acad Sci USA 48:9–16, 1962.

52. Davidson, RG, Nitowsky, HM & Childs, B. Demonstration of two populations of cells in the human female heterozygous for glucose-6-phosphate dehydrogenase variants. Proc Natl Acad Sci USA 50:481–485, 1963.

53. Beutler, E. G6PD: population genetics and clinical manifestations. Blood Rev 10:45–52, 1996.

54. Tishkoff, SA, Varkonyi, R, Cahinhinan, N, Abbes, S, Argyropoulos, G, Destro-Bisol, G, et al. Haplotype diversity and linkage disequilibrium at human G6PD: recent origin of alleles that confer malarial resistance. Science 293:455–462, 2001.

55. Siniscalco, M, Latte, B & Motulsky, AG. Favism and thalassemia in Sardinia and their relationship to malaria. Nature 190:1179–1180, 1961.

56. Ganczakowski, M, Town, M, Bowden, DK, Vulliamy, TJ, Kaneko, A, Clegg, JB, et al. Multiple glucose 6-phosphate

dehydrogenase-deficient variants correlate with malaria ende-
micity in the Vanuatu archipelago (southwestern Pacific). Am J
Hum Genet 56:294–301, 1995.

57. Szeinberg, A, Sheba, C & Adam, A. Selective occurrence of glutathione instability in red corpuscles of the various Jewish tribes.
Blood 13:1043–1053, 1958.

58. Bonne, B. Chaim Sheba (1908–1971). Am J Phys Anthropol
36:311–313, 1972.

59. Sheba, C, Szeinberg, A, Ramot, B, Adam, A & Ashkenazi, I.
Epidemiologic surveys of deleterious genes in different population groups in Israel. Am J Public Health 52:1101–1106, 1962.

60. Comings, DE. In Memoriam: Richard M. Goodman, M.D.
Am J Med Genet 38:517, 1991.

61. McKusick, VA. Ethnic distribution of disease in non-Jews.
Isr J Med Sci 9:1375–1382, 1973.

62. McKusick, VA. *Mendelian Inheritance in Man*, (Johns Hopkins
University Press, Baltimore, 1998).

63. Goodman, RM. *Genetic Disorders Among Jewish People*, (Johns Hopkins
University Press, Baltimore, 1979).

64. Buerger, L. Thrombo-angiitis obliterans: A study of the vascular
lesions leading to presenile spontaneous gangrene. Am J Med Sci
136:567–580, 1908.

65. Olin, JW & Shih, A. Thromboangiitis obliterans (Buerger's disease). Curr Opin Rheumatol 18:18–24, 2006.

66. Goodman, RM, Adam, A & Sheba, C. A genetic study of stub
thumbs among various ethnic groups in Israel. J Med Genet
39:116–121, 1965.

67. Goodman, RM. Various genetic traits and diseases among the
Jewish ethnic groups. Birth Defects Orig Artic Ser 10:205–219,
1974.

68. Tay, W. Symmetric changes in the region of the yellow spot in each eye of an infant. Trans Ophthalmol Soc UK 1:55–57, 1881.

69. Sachs, B. On arrested cerebral development with special reference to its cortical pathology. J Nervous Mental Disease 14:541–553, 1887.

70. Sachs, B. A familial form of idiocy, generally fatal, associated with early blindness (amaurotic familial idiocy). J Nervous Mental Disease 21:475–479, 1896.

71. Kaback, M, Lim-Steele, J, Dabholkar, D, Brown, D, Levy, N & Zeiger, K. Tay-Sachs disease—carrier screening, prenatal diagnosis, and the molecular era. An international perspective, 1970 to 1993. The International TSD Data Collection Network. JAMA 270:2307–2315, 1993.

72. Kaback, MM. Screening and prevention in Tay-Sachs disease: origins, update, and impact. Adv Genet 44:253–265, 2001.

73. Kaback, MM, Nathan, TJ & Greenwald, S. Tay-Sachs disease: heterozygote screening and prenatal diagnosis—U.S. experience and world perspective. Prog Clin Biol Res 18:13–36, 1977.

74. Myrianthopoulos, NC & Aronson, SM. Population dynamics of Tay-Sachs disease. I. Reproductive fitness and selection. Am J Hum Genet 18:313–327, 1966.

75. Myrianthopoulos, NC & Melnick, M. Tay-Sachs disease: a genetic-historical view of selective advantage. Prog Clin Biol Res 18:95–106, 1977.

76. Mayr, E. *Animal Species and Evolution*, (Belknap Press, Cambridge, MA, 1965).

77. Chase, GA & McKusick, VA. Controversy in human genetics: founder effect in Tay-Sachs disease. Am J Hum Genet 24:339–340, 1972.

78. Stevens, RF. The history of haemophilia in the royal families of Europe. Br J Haematol 105:25–32, 1999.

79. Ostrer, H. A genetic profile of contemporary Jewish populations. Nat Rev Genet 2:891–898, 2001.

80. Yepiskoposyan, L & Harutyunyan, A. Population genetics of familial Mediterranean fever: a review. Eur J Hum Genet 15:911–916, 2007.

81. John, EM, Miron, A, Gong, G, Phipps, AI, Felberg, A, Li, FP, et al. Prevalence of pathogenic BRCA1 mutation carriers in 5 US racial/ethnic groups. JAMA 298:2869–2876, 2007.

81a. Velez, C, Palamara, PF, Guevara-Aguirre, J, Hao, L, Karafet, T, Guevara-Aguirre, M, et al. The impact of Converso Jews on the genomes of modern Latin Americans. Hum Genet 131:251–63, 2012.

82. Brunt, PW & McKusick, VA. Familial dysautonomia. A report of genetic and clinical studies, with a review of the literature. Medicine (Baltimore) 49:343–374, 1970.

83. Blumenfeld, A, Slaugenhaupt, SA, Liebert, CB, Temper, V, Maayan, C, Gill, S, et al. Precise genetic mapping and haplotype analysis of the familial dysautonomia gene on human chromosome 9q31. Am J Hum Genet 64:1110–1118, 1999.

84. Risch, N, Tang, H, Katzenstein, H & Ekstein, J. Geographic distribution of disease mutations in the Ashkenazi Jewish population supports genetic drift over selection. Am J Hum Genet 72:812–822, 2003.

85. Slaugenhaupt, SA, Acierno, JS, Jr., Helbling, LA, Bove, C, Goldin, E, Bach, G, et al. Mapping of the mucolipidosis type IV gene to chromosome 19p and definition of founder haplotypes. Am J Hum Genet 65:773–778, 1999.

86. Ellis, NA, Ciocci, S, Proytcheva, M, Lennon, D, Groden, J & German, J. The Ashkenazic Jewish Bloom syndrome mutation

blmAsh is present in non-Jewish Americans of Spanish ancestry. Am J Hum Genet 63:1685–1693, 1998.

87. Goldstein, DB, Reich, DE, Bradman, N, Usher, S, Seligsohn, U & Peretz, H. Age estimates of two common mutations causing factor XI deficiency: recent genetic drift is not necessary for elevated disease incidence among Ashkenazi Jews. Am J Hum Genet 64:1071–1075, 1999.

88. Zabetian, CP, Hutter, CM, Yearout, D, Lopez, AN, Factor, SA, Griffith, A, et al. LRRK2 G2019S in families with Parkinson disease who originated from Europe and the Middle East: evidence of two distinct founding events beginning two millennia ago. Am J Hum Genet 79:752–758, 2006.

89. Ben-Yosef, T, Ness, SL, Madeo, AC, Bar-Lev, A, Wolfman, JH, Ahmed, ZM, et al. A mutation of PCDH15 among Ashkenazi Jews with the type 1 Usher syndrome. N Engl J Med 348:1664–1670, 2003.

90. Diaz, GA, Gelb, BD, Risch, N, Nygaard, TG, Frisch, A, Cohen, IJ, et al. Gaucher disease: the origins of the Ashkenazi Jewish N370S and 84GG acid beta-glucosidase mutations. Am J Hum Genet 66:1821–1832, 2000.

91. Durst, R, Colombo, R, Shpitzen, S, Avi, LB, Friedlander, Y, Wexler, R, et al. Recent origin and spread of a common Lithuanian mutation, G197del LDLR, causing familial hypercholesterolemia: positive selection is not always necessary to account for disease incidence among Ashkenazi Jews. Am J Hum Genet 68:1172–1188, 2001.

92. Blumen, SC, Korczyn, AD, Lavoie, H, Medynski, S, Chapman, J, Asherov, A, et al. Oculopharyngeal muscular dystrophy among Bukhara Jews is due to a founder (GCG)9 mutation in the PABP2 gene. Neurology 55:1267–1270, 2000.

93. Chouraqui, AN. *Between East and West: A History of the Jews of North Africa*, (Jewish Publication Society, Philadelphia, 1969).

94. Morell, RJ, Kim, HJ, Hood, LJ, Goforth, L, Friderici, K, Fisher, R, et al. Mutations in the Connexin 26 gene (GJB2) among Ashkenazi Jews with nonsyndromic recessive deafness. N Engl J Med 339:1500–1505, 1998.

95. Kaufman, M, Grinshpun-Cohen, J, Karpati, M, Peleg, L, Goldman, B, Akstein, E, et al. Tay-Sachs disease and HEXA mutations among Moroccan Jews. Hum Mutat 10:295–300, 1997.

96. Zlotogora, J. High frequencies of human genetic diseases: founder effect with genetic drift or selection? Am J Med Genet 49:10–13, 1994.

97. Motulsky, AG, Vandepitte, J & Fraser, GR. Population genetic studies in the Congo. I. Glucose-6-phosphate dehydrogenase deficiency, hemoglobin S, and malaria. Am J Hum Genet 18:514–537, 1966.

98. Allison, AC. Protection afforded by sickle-cell trait against subtertian malareal infection. Br Med J 1:290–294, 1954.

99. Cuthbert, AW, Halstead, J, Ratcliff, R, Colledge, WH & Evans, MJ. The genetic advantage hypothesis in cystic fibrosis heterozygotes: a murine study. J Physiol 482:449–454, 1995.

100. Efron, JM. *Defenders of the Race: Jewish Doctors and Race Science in Fin-de-Siècle Europe*, (Yale University Press, New Haven, 1994).

101. Benjamin, D. Joseph Jacobs. Australian Jewish Historical Society 3:72–91, 1949.

102. Marx, A. *Essays in Jewish Biography*, (Jewish Publication Society of America, Philadelphia, 1947).

103. Jacobs, J. *Jewish Ideals, and Other Essays*, xviii, 242 p. (Books for Libraries Press, Freeport, NY, 1972).

104. Eliot, G. *Daniel Deronda*, 2 v. (Harper & Brothers, New York, 1876).

105. Holmstrom, J & Lerner, L. *George Eliot and Her Readers; A Selection of Contemporary Reviews*, 190 p. (Barnes & Noble, New York, 1966).

106. Galton, F. Types and their inheritance. Nature 32:507–510, 1885.

107. Skorecki, K, Selig, S, Blazer, S, Bradman, R, Bradman, N, Waburton, PJ, et al. Y chromosomes of Jewish priests. Nature 385:32, 1997.

108. Thomas, MG, Skorecki, K, Ben-Ami, H, Parfitt, T, Bradman, N & Goldstein, DB. Origins of old testament priests. Nature 394:138–140, 1998.

109. Executive Committee of the Editorial Board, & Jacobs, J. Cohen. in *The Jewish Encyclopedia*, Vol. 4, 144 p. ed. Adler, C. Funk and Wagnell's, New York, 1906.

110. Bradman, N, Thomas, MG & Goldstein, D. The genetic origins of Old Testament priests. in *Population specific polymorphisms.* ed. Renfrew, C.E. 31–44 p. (Cambridge University Press, Cambridge, United Kingdom, 1999).

111. Mitchell, RJ & Hammer, MF. Human evolution and the Y chromosome. Curr Opin Genet Dev 6:737–742, 1996.

112. Underhill, PA, Jin, L, Lin, AA, Mehdi, SQ, Jenkins, T, Vollrath, D, et al. Detection of numerous Y chromosome biallelic polymorphisms by denaturing high-performance liquid chromatography. Genome Res 7:996–1005, 1997.

113. Karafet, TM, Mendez, FL, Meilerman, MB, Underhill, PA, Zegura, SL & Hammer, MF. New binary polymorphisms reshape and increase resolution of the human Y chromosomal haplogroup tree. Genome Res 18:830–838, 2008.

114. Semino, O, Magri, C, Benuzzi, G, Lin, AA, Al-Zahery, N, Battaglia, V, et al. Origin, diffusion, and differentiation of Y-chromosome

haplogroups E and J: inferences on the neolithization of Europe and later migratory events in the Mediterranean area. Am J Hum Genet 74:1023–1034, 2004.

115. Walsh, B. Estimating the time to the most recent common ancestor for the Y chromosome or mitochondrial DNA for a pair of individuals. Genetics 158:897–912, 2001.

116. Hammer, MF, Redd, AJ, Wood, ET, Bonner, MR, Jarjanazi, H, Karafet, T, et al. Jewish and Middle Eastern non-Jewish populations share a common pool of Y-chromosome biallelic haplotypes. Proc Natl Acad Sci USA 97:6769–6774, 2000.

117. Behar, DM, Garrigan, D, Kaplan, ME, Mobasher, Z, Rosengarten, D, Karafet, TM, et al. Contrasting patterns of Y chromosome variation in Ashkenazi Jewish and host non-Jewish European populations. Hum Genet 114:354–365, 2004.

118. Semino, O, Passarino, G, Oefner, PJ, Lin, AA, Arbuzova, S, Beckman, LE, De Benedictis, G, et al. The genetic legacy of Paleolithic Homo sapiens sapiens in extant Europeans: a Y chromosome perspective. Science 290:1155–1159, 2000.

119. Nebel, A, Filon, D, Brinkmann, B, Majumder, PP, Faerman, M & Oppenheim, A. The Y chromosome pool of Jews as part of the genetic landscape of the Middle East. Am J Hum Genet 69:1095–1112, 2001.

120. Nebel, A, Filon, D, Faerman, M, Soodyall, H & Oppenheim, A. Y chromosome evidence for a founder effect in Ashkenazi Jews. Eur J Hum Genet 13:388–391, 2005.

121. Zalloua, PA, Xue, Y, Khalife, J, Makhoul, N, Debiane, L, Platt, DE, et al. Y-chromosomal diversity in Lebanon is structured by recent historical events. Am J Hum Genet 82:873–882, 2008.

122. Entine, J. *Abraham's Children: Race, Identity, and the DNA of the Chosen People*, xi, 420 p. (Grand Central Pub, New York, 2007).

123. Goldstein, DB. *Jacob's legacy: a genetic view of Jewish history*, xvii, 148 p. (Yale University Press, New Haven, CT, 2008).

124. Cruciani, F, La Fratta, R, Santolamazza, P, Sellitto, D, Pascone, R, Moral, P, et al. Phylogeographic analysis of haplogroup E3b (E-M215) y chromosomes reveals multiple migratory events within and out of Africa. Am J Hum Genet 74:1014–1022, 2004.

125. Ekins, JE, Tinah, EN, Myres, NM, Ritchie, KH, Perego, UA, Ekins, JB, et al. An updated world-wide characterization of the Cohen Modal Haplotype. American Society of Human Genetics 2005 meeting, Salt Lake City Utah. Poster #1045 (http://www.smgf.org/resources/papers/ASHG2005_Jayne.pdf).

126. Hammer, MF, Behar, DM, Karafet, TM, Mendez, FL, Hallmark, B, Erez, T, et al. Extended Y chromosome haplotypes resolve multiple and unique lineages of the Jewish priesthood. Hum Genet 126:707–717, 2009.

127. Thomas, MG, Parfitt, T, Weiss, DA, Skorecki, K, Wilson, JF, le Roux, M, et al. Y chromosomes traveling south: the cohen modal haplotype and the origins of the Lemba—the Black Jews of Southern Africa. Am J Hum Genet 66:674–686, 2000.

128. NOVA online. The Lemba, The Black Jews of Southern Africa. 2000 (http://www.pbs.org/wgbh/nova/israel/familylemba.html).

129. Parfitt, T & Egorova, Y. *Genetics, Mass Media and Identity: A Case Study of the Genetic Research on the Lemba and Bene Israel*, 150 p. (Routledge, London; New York, 2006).

130. Behar, DM, Thomas, MG, Skorecki, K, Hammer, MF, Bulygina, E, Rosengarten, D, et al. Multiple origins of Ashkenazi Levites: Y chromosome evidence for both Near Eastern and European ancestries. Am J Hum Genet 73:768–779, 2003.

131. Cavalli-Sforza, LL, Menozzi, P & Piazza, A. *The History and Geography of Human Genes*, xi, 541, 518 p. (Princeton University Press, Princeton, NJ, 1994).

132. Lehmann, MB. *Ladino Rabbinic Literature and Ottoman Sephardic Culture*, viii, 264 p. (Indiana University Press, Bloomington, IN, 2005).

133. Gottheil, R & Wiener, L. Judaeo-German. in *Jewish Encyclopedia*, Vol. 7, 307–309 p. ed. Adler, C. Funk and Wagnalls, New York, 1906.

134. Wexler, P. *Two-Tiered Relexification in Yiddish: Jews, Sorbs, Khazars, and the Kiev-Polessian Dialect*, (Mouton de Gruyter, Berlin, and New York, 2002).

136. Biran, A & Naveh, J. An Aramaic stele fragment from Tel Dan. Israel Explor J 43:81–98, 1993.

137. Menton, AF. *The Book of Destiny*, xi, 611 p. (King David Press, Cold Spring Harbor, NY, 1996).

138. Shaltiel, M. http://www.shaltiel.com. 2007.

139. Cann, RL, Stoneking, M & Wilson, AC. Mitochondrial DNA and human evolution. Nature 325:31–36, 1987.

140. Wilson, AC & Cann, RL. The recent African genesis of humans. Sci Am 266:68–73, 1992.

141. Patterson, N, Richter, DJ, Gnerre, S, Lander, ES & Reich, D. Genetic evidence for complex speciation of humans and chimpanzees. Nature 441:1103–1108, 2006.

142. Cox, MP, Mendez, FL, Karafet, TM, Pilkington, MM, Kingan, SB, Destro-Bisol, G, et al. Testing for archaic hominin admixture on the X chromosome: model likelihoods for the modern human RRM2P4 region from summaries of genealogical topology under the structured coalescent. Genetics 178:427–437, 2008.

143. Behar, DM, Metspalu, E, Kivisild, T, Achilli, A, Hadid, Y, Tzur, S, et al. The matrilineal ancestry of Ashkenazi Jewry: portrait of a recent founder event. Am J Hum Genet 78:487–497, 2006.

144. Behar, DM, Metspalu, E, Kivisild, T, Rosset, S, Tzur, S, Hadid, Y, et al. Counting the founders: the matrilineal genetic ancestry of the Jewish Diaspora. PLoS One 3:e2062, 2008.

145. Benjamin of Tudela. *The Itinerary of Benjamin of Tudela: Travels in the Middle Ages*, 169 p. (J. Simon, Malibu, CA, 1983).

146. Thomas, MG, Weale, ME, Jones, AL, Richards, M, Smith, A, Redhead, N, et al. Founding mothers of Jewish communities: geographically separated Jewish groups were independently founded by very few female ancestors. Am J Hum Genet 70:1411–1420, 2002.

147. Wells, S. *Deep Ancestry: Inside the Genographic Project*, 247 p. (National Geographic, Washington, D.C., 2006).

148. Behar, DM, Villems, R, Soodyall, H, Blue-Smith, J, Pereira, L, Metspalu, E, et al. The dawn of human matrilineal diversity. Am J Hum Genet 82:1130–1140, 2008.

149. Mourant, AE, Kopeâc, AC & Domaniewska-Sobczak, K. *The Genetics of the Jews*, vi, 122 p. (Clarendon Press, Oxford [Eng.]; New York, 1978).

150. Roberts, DF. Obituary: Arthur Mourant (1904–1994). Human Biology 69:277–289, 1997.

151. Landsteiner, K. On individual differences in human blood. in *Nobel Lectures, Physiology or Medicine 1922–1941*, Elsevier Publishing Company, Amsterdam, 1965. "Karl Landsteiner - Nobel Lecture". Nobelprize.org. 17 Dec 2011 http://www.nobelprize.org/nobel_prizes/medicine/laureates/1930/landsteiner-lecture.html

152. Mourant, AE. *The ABO Blood Groups; Comprehensive Tables and Maps of World Distribution*, viii, 276 p. (Blackwell Scientific Publications, Oxford [Eng.], 1958).

153. Mourant, AE, Kopec, AC & Domaniewska-Sobczak, K. *The Distribution of the Human Blood Groups, and Other Polymorphisms*, xiv, 1055 p., 13 leaves of plates (Oxford University Press, London, 1976).

154. Etcheverry, MA. El factor rhesus: su genética e importancia clínica. El Día Médico 17:1237–1259, 1945.

155. Landsteiner, K & Wiener, AS. Studies on an agglutinogen (Rh) in human blood reacting with anti-Rhesus sera and with human isoantibodies. J Exp Med 74:309–320, 1941.

156. Levine, P, Vogel, P, Katzin, EM & Burnham, L. Pathogenesis of erythroblastosis fetalis: statistical evidence. Science 94:371–372, 1941.

157. Landsteiner, K & Levine, P. On the inheritance of agglutinogens of human blood demonstrable by immune agglutinins. J Exp Med 48:731–749, 1928.

158. Pollack, W, Gorman, JG, Freda, VJ, Ascari, WQ, Allen, AE & Baker, WJ. Results of clinical trials of RhoGAM in women. Transfusion 8:151–153, 1968.

159. Parfitt, T. *The Lost Tribes of Israel: The History of a Myth*, 277 p., 8 p. of plates (Weidenfeld & Nicolson, London, 2002).

160. Cavalli-Sforza, LL & Cavalli-Sforza, F. *The Great Human Diasporas: The History of Diversity and Evolution*, xiii, 300 p. (Addison-Wesley, Reading, Mass., 1995).

161. Fisher, RA. *The Genetical Theory of Natural Selection*, xiv, 272 p. (The Clarendon Press, Oxford, 1930).

162. Cavalli-Sforza, LL & Edwards, AW. Phylogenetic analysis. Models and estimation procedures. Am J Hum Genet 19:233–257, 1967.

163. Edwards, AW & Cavalli-Sforza, LL. A method for cluster analysis. Biometrics 21:362–375, 1965.

164. Carmelli, D & Cavalli-Sforza, LL. The genetic origin of the Jews: a multivariate approach. Hum Biol 51:41–61, 1979.

165. Rao, DC & Morton, NE. Large deviations in the distribution of rare genes. Am J Hum Genet 25:594–597, 1973.

166. Bonne-Tamir, B, Bodmer, JG, Bodmer, WF, Pickbourne, P, Brautbar, C, Gazit, E, et al. HLA polymorphism in Israel. 9. An overall comparative analysis. Tissue Antigens 11:235–250, 1978.

167. Karlin, S, Kenett, R & Bonne-Tamir, B. Analysis of biochemical genetic data on Jewish populations: II. Results and interpretations of heterogeneity indices and distance measures with respect to standards. Am J Hum Genet 31:341–365, 1979.

168. Kobyliansky, E, Micle, S, Goldschmidt-Nathan, M, Arensburg, B & Nathan, H. Jewish populations of the world: genetic likeness and differences. Ann Hum Biol 9:1–34, 1982.

169. Livshits, G, Sokal, RR & Kobyliansky, E. Genetic affinities of Jewish populations. Am J Hum Genet 49:131–146, 1991.

170. Wijsman, EM. Techniques for estimating genetic admixture and applications to the problem of the origin of the Icelanders and the Ashkenazi Jews. Hum Genet 67:441–448, 1984.

171. Bonne-Tamir, B, Ashbel, S & Bar-Shani, S. Ethnic communities in Israel: the genetic blood markers of the Babylonian Jews. Am J Phys Anthropol 49:457–464, 1978.

172. Patai, R & Patai-Wing, J. *The Myth of the Jewish Race*, (Scribner, New York, 1975).

173. Venter, JC, Adams, MD, Myers, EW, Li, PW, Mural, RJ, Sutton, GG, et al. The sequence of the human genome. Science 291:1304–1351, 2001.

174. Lander, ES, Linton, LM, Birren, B, Nusbaum, C, Zody, MC, Baldwin, J, et al. Initial sequencing and analysis of the human genome. Nature 409:860–921, 2001.

175. Redon, R, Ishikawa, S, Fitch, KR, Feuk, L, Perry, GH, Andrews, TD, et al. Global variation in copy number in the human genome. Nature 444:444–454, 2006.

176. Li, JZ, Absher, DM, Tang, H, Southwick, AM, Casto, AM, Ramachandran, S, et al. Worldwide human relationships inferred from genome-wide patterns of variation. Science 319:1100–1104, 2008.

177. A comprehensive genetic linkage map of the human genome. NIH/CEPH Collaborative Mapping Group. Science 258:67–86, 1992.

178. Pritchard, JK, Stephens, M & Donnelly, P. Inference of population structure using multilocus genotype data. Genetics 155:945–959, 2000.

179. Rosenberg, NA, Pritchard, JK, Weber, JL, Cann, HM, Kidd, KK, Zhivotovsky, LA et al. Genetic structure of human populations. Science 298:2381–2385, 2002.

180. Rosenberg, NA, Woolf, E, Pritchard, JK, Schaap, T, Gefel, D, Shpirer, I, et al. Distinctive genetic signatures in the Libyan Jews. Proc Natl Acad Sci USA 98:858–863, 2001.

181. Bonne-Tamir, B, Ashbel, S & Modai, J. Genetic markers in Libyan Jews. Hum Genet 37:319–28, 1977.

182. De Felice, R. *Jews in an Arab Land: Libya, 1835–1970*, x, 406 p., 16 p. of plates (University of Texas Press, Austin, TX, 1985).

183. Neugut, RH, Neugut, AI, Kahana, E, Stein, Z & Alter, M. Creutzfeldt-Jakob disease: familial clustering among Libyan-born Israelis. Neurology 29:225–231, 1979.

184. Colombo, R. Age and origin of the PRNP E200K mutation causing familial Creutzfeldt-Jacob disease in Libyan Jews. Am J Hum Genet 67:528–531, 2000.

185. International Human HapMap Consortium. A haplotype map of the human genome. Nature 437:1299–1320, 2005.

186. Newman, MEJ, Barabási, A-L & Watts, DJ. *The Structure and Dynamics of Networks,* x, 582 p. (Princeton University Press, Princeton, NJ, 2006).

187. Novembre, J, Johnson, T, Bryc, K, Kutalik, Z, Boyko, AR, Auton, A, et al. Genes mirror geography within Europe. Nature 456:98–101, 2008.

188. Price, AL, Butler, J, Patterson, N, Capelli, C, Pascali, VL, Scarnicci, F, et al. Discerning the ancestry of European Americans in genetic association studies. PLoS Genet 4:e236, 2008.

189. Seldin, MF, Shigeta, R, Villoslada, P, Selmi, C, Tuomilehto, J, Silva, G, et al. European population substructure: clustering of northern and southern populations. PLoS Genet 2:e143, 2006.

190. Need, AC, Kasperaviciute, D, Cirulli, ET & Goldstein, DB. A genome-wide genetic signature of Jewish ancestry perfectly separates individuals with and without full Jewish ancestry in a large random sample of European Americans. Genome Biol 10:R7, 2009.

191. Oddoux, C, Guillen-Navarro, E, Ditivoli, C, Dicave, E, Cilio, MR, Clayton, CM, et al. Mendelian diseases among Roman Jews: implications for the origins of disease alleles. J Clin Endocrinol Metab 84:4405–4409, 1999.

192. Shorto, R. *The Island at the Center of the World: the Epic Story of Dutch Manhattan and the Forgotten Colony that Shaped America,* xiv, 384 p. (Doubleday, New York, 2004).

193. Baron, SW. *Social and Religious History of the Jews,* (Columbia University Press, New York, 1937).

194. Roth, C. *The History of the Jews of Italy,* (Jewish Publication Society of America, Philadelphia, 1946).

195.   Curtis, M, Neyer, J, Waxman, CI & Pollack, A. *The Palestinians: People History, Politics*, (Transaction Books, New Brunswick, NJ, 1975).

196.   Falah, SH. *The Druzes in the Middle East*, (Druze Research and Publication Institute, New York, 2002).

197.   Kay, S. *The Bedouin*, (Crane, Russak & Company, New York, 1978).

198.   Galton, F. *Hereditary Genius: An Inquiry into its Laws and Consequences*, vi, 2 390 p. (Macmillan and co., London, 1869).

199.   Darwin, C. *The Variation of Animals and Plants under Domestication*, 2 v. (O. Judd & company, New York,, 1868).

200.   Jacobs, J. *Jewish Contributions to Civilization: An Estimate*, 334 p. (The Jewish Publication Society of America, Philadelphia, 1919).

201.   Hughes, A. Jews and Gentiles: Their intellectual and tempermental differences. Eugenics Rev 18:1–6, 1928.

202.   Kamin, LJ. *The Science and Politics of I.Q*, vii, 183 p. (L. Erlbaum Associates; distributed by Halsted Press, New York, Potomac, Md., 1974).

203.   Franklin, A. *Ending the Mendel-Fisher Controversy*, x, 330 p. (University of Pittsburgh Press, Pittsburgh, PA, 2008).

204.   Gillie, O. Crucial data was faked by eminent psychologist. In *Sunday Times*, London, 1976.

205.   Gould, SJ. *The Mismeasure of Man*, 352 p. (Norton, New York, 1981).

206.   Murray, C. Jewish genius. In *Commentary Magazine*, April, 2007. http://www.commentarymagazine.com/article/jewish-genius/

207.   Herrnstein, RJ & Murray, CA. *The Bell Curve: Intelligence and Class Structure in American Life*, xxvi, 845 p. (Free Press, New York, 1994).

208.   Cochran, G, Hardy, J & Harpending, H. Natural history of Ashkenazi intelligence. J Biosoc Sci 38:659–693, 2006.

209.   Dershowitz, AM. *The Vanishing American Jew: In Search of Jewish Identity for the Next Century*, x, 395 p. (Little, Brown, Boston, 1997).

210. Singer, IB. The art of fiction. In *Paris Review*, 1988.

211. Senior, J. Are Jews smarter? in *New York Magazine*, 2005.

212. Ortar, GR. Educational achievements of primary school graduates in Israel as related to their socio-cultural background. Comparative Education 4:23–34, 1967.

213. Flynn, JR. *What is Intelligence?: Beyond the Flynn Effect*, xi, 216 p. (Cambridge University Press, Cambridge, UK; New York, 2007).

214. Fraser, S. *The Bell Curve Wars: Race, Intelligence, and the Future of America*, vi, 216 p. (BasicBooks, New York, 1995).

215. Rodrigue, A. *Images of Sephardi and Eastern Jewries in Transition: The Teachers of the Alliance Israélite Universelle, 1860–1939*, ix, 308 p. (University of Washington Press, Seattle, WA, 1993).

216. Alliance Israélite Universelle. *Annual Report of the Alliance Israélite Universelle*, (Offices of the Society, Paris, 1885).

217. Roden, C. *The Book of Jewish Food: an Odyssey from Samarkand to New York*, xiv, 668 p. (Knopf: Distrubuted by Random House, New York, 1996).

218. Gladwell, M. *Outliers : The Story of Success*, 309 p. (Little, Brown and Co., New York, 2008).

219. Rhodes, R. *The Making of the Atomic Bomb*, 886 p., 42 p. of plates (Simon & Schuster, New York, 1986).

220. de Sola Price, DJ. *Little Science, Big Science*, 119 p. (Columbia University Press, New York,, 1963).

221. Galton, F. The history of twins, as a criterion of the relative power of nature and nurture. In *Fraser's Magazine* Vol. 12 566–576, 1875.

222. Klein, RJ, Zeiss, C, Chew, EY, Tsai, JY, Sackler, RS, Haynes, C, et al. Complement factor H polymorphism in age-related macular degeneration. Science 308:385–389, 2005.

223. Butcher, LM, Davis, OS, Craig, IW & Plomin, R. Genome-wide quantitative trait locus association scan of general cognitive ability using pooled DNA and 500K single nucleotide polymorphism microarrays. Genes Brain Behav 7:435–446, 2008.

224. Kohn, R & Levav, I. Jews and their intraethnic differential vulnerability to affective disorders, fact or artifact? I: An overview of the literature. Isr J Psychiatry Relat Sci 31:261–270, 1994.

225. Kohn, R, Levav, I, Dohrenwend, BP, Shrout, PE & Skodol, AE. Jews and their intraethnic vulnerability to affective disorders, fact or artifact? II: Evidence from a cohort study. Isr J Psychiatry Relat Sci 34:149–156, 1997.

226. Levav, I, Kohn, R, Golding, JM & Weissman, MM. Vulnerability of Jews to affective disorders. Am J Psychiatry 154:941–947, 1997.

227. Fallin, MD, Lasseter, VK, Wolyniec, PS, McGrath, JA, Nestadt, G, Valle, D, et al. Genomewide linkage scan for bipolar-disorder susceptibility loci among Ashkenazi Jewish families. Am J Hum Genet 75:204–219, 2004.

228. Kieseppa, T, Partonen, T, Haukka, J, Kaprio, J & Lonnqvist, J. High concordance of bipolar I disorder in a nationwide sample of twins. Am J Psychiatry 161:1814–1821, 2004.

229. Taylor, L, Faraone, SV & Tsuang, MT. Family, twin, and adoption studies of bipolar disease. Curr Psychiatry Rep 4:130–133, 2002.

230. Roy, A, Nielsen, D, Rylander, G, Sarchiapone, M & Segal, N. Genetics of suicide in depression. J Clin Psychiatry 60 Suppl 2:12–7; discussion 18–20, 113–116, 1999.

231. Jamison, KR. *Night Falls Fast: Understanding Suicide*, x, 432 p. (Knopf, New York, 1999).

232. Weissman, MM, Wickramaratne, P, Nomura, Y, Warner, V, Pilowsky, D & Verdeli, H. Offspring of depressed parents: 20 years later. Am J Psychiatry 163:1001–1008, 2006.

233. Pulver, AE, Sawyer, JW & Childs, B. The association between season of birth and the risk for schizophrenia. Am J Epidemiol 114:735–749, 1981.

234. Avramopoulos, D, Lasseter, VK, Fallin, MD, Wolyniec, PS, McGrath, JA, Nestadt, G, et al. Stage II follow-up on a linkage scan for bipolar disorder in the Ashkenazim provides suggestive evidence for chromosome 12p and the GRIN2B gene. Genet Med 9:745–751, 2007.

235. Shifman, S, Bronstein, M, Sternfeld, M, Pisante-Shalom, A, Lev-Lehman, E, Weizman, A, et al. A highly significant association between a COMT haplotype and schizophrenia. Am J Hum Genet 71:1296–1302, 2002.

236. Post, F. Creativity and psychopathology. A study of 291 world-famous men. Br J Psychiatry 165:22–34, 1994.

237. Schildkraut, JJ, Hirshfeld, AJ & Murphy, JM. Mind and mood in modern art, II: Depressive disorders, spirituality, and early deaths in the abstract expressionist artists of the New York School. Am J Psychiatry 151:482–488, 1994.

238. Jamison, KR. *Touched with Fire: Manic-Depressive Illness and the Artistic Temperament*, xii, 370 p. (Free Press; Maxwell Macmillan Canada; Maxwell Macmillan International, New York; Toronto, 1993).

239. Dorff, EN. *Matters of Life and Death: a Jewish Approach to Modern Medical Ethics*, xix, 456 p. (Jewish Publication Society, Philadelphia, 1998).

240. Charrow, J. Enzyme replacement therapy for Gaucher disease. Expert Opin Biol Ther 9:121–131, 2009.

241.   Robson, M & Offit, K. Clinical practice. Management of an inherited predisposition to breast cancer. N Engl J Med 357:154–162, 2007.

242.   Maddox, B. *Rosalind Franklin: the Dark Lady of DNA*, xix, 380 p., 16 p. of plates (HarperCollins, New York, 2002).

243.   Rubinstein, WS, Jiang, H, Dellefave, L & Rademaker, AW. Cost-effectiveness of population-based BRCA1/2 testing and ovarian cancer prevention for Ashkenazi Jews: a call for dialogue. Genet Med 11:629–639, 2009.

244.   Levy-Lahad, E. Population-based BRCA1/BRCA2 screening in Ashkenazi Jews: a call for evidence. Genet Med 11:620–621, 2009.

245.   Breast Cancer Research Foundation,2008. http://www.bcrfcure.org/action_0708grantees_levylahad.html. December 17, 2011.

246.   National Human Genome Research Institute. http://www.genome.gov/12010659, December 17, 2011.

247.   Isaacson, W. How Einstein divided America's Jews. In *The Atlantic*, 2009.

248.   Isaacson, W. *Einstein: His Life and Universe*, xxii, 675, 16 p. of plates (Simon & Schuster, New York, 2007).

249.   Einstein, A & Harris, A. *The World as I See It*, xvi p., 1 l., (Covici, Friede, New York, 1934).

250.   Einstein, A. *The Collected Papers of Albert Einstein: Correspondence, January-December 1921 [English translation]*, (Princeton University Press, Princeton, NJ, 2009).

251.   Novick, P. *The Holocaust in American Life*, 373 p. (Houghton Mifflin, Boston, 1999).

252.   An Act To Amend The Education Law, In Relation To Instruction On Subjects Of Human Rights Violations, Genocide, Slavery, And The Holocaust. in *S7765* ed. Legislature, N.Y.S., 1994.

253.   An Act to Create The Mississippi Commission On the Holocaust; To Provide For The Membership Of The Commission;

To Provide For the Powers and Duties Of The Commission; And For Related Purposes. Vol. 1269 ed. Mississippi, 2004.

254. United States Holocaust Memorial Museum, 1984 http://www. ushmm.org/remembrance/dor/. December 17, 2011.

255. Berr, H & Bellos, D. *The Journal of Hélène Berr*, 307 p. (Weinstein Books, New York., 2008).

256. Dawidowicz, LS. *The War Against the Jews, 1933–1945*, xviii, 460 p. (Holt, Rinehart and Winston, New York, 1975).

257. Hobson, LKZ. *Gentleman's Agreement: A Novel*, 275 p. (Simon and Schuster, New York, 1947).

258. Gladwell, M. *Outliers: The Story of Success*, (Little, Brown and Co., New York, NY, 2008).

259. American Jewish Year Book. v. American Jewish Committee, Philadelphia, 2007.

260. Silberman, CE. *A Certain People: American Jews and their Lives Today*, 458 p. (Summit Books, New York, 1985).

261. Hertzberg, A. The triumph of the Jews. In *New York Review of Books*, 1985.

262. Goodman, W. Books of the Times. In *New York Times*, 1985.

263. Gessen, M. *Blood Matters: From Inherited Illness to Designer Babies, How the World and I Found Ourselves in the Future of the Gene*, 321 p. (Harcourt, Orlando, FL, 2008).

264. Simon, G. *Nationalism and Policy Toward the Nationalities in the Soviet Union: From Totalitarian Dictatorship to Post-Stalinist Society*, xvii, 483 p. (Westview Press, Boulder, CO, 1991).

265. Israel. & Aryeh Greenfield-A.G. Publications (Israel). *Israel's written constitution: verbatim English translations of the Declaration of Independence and of the Basic Laws, consolidated and updated as of January 10, 1999*, 80 p. (Aryeh Greenfield—A.G. Publications, Haifa, 1999).

266. Gouldman, MD. *Israel Nationality Law*, 151 p. (Institute for Legislative Research and Comparative Law, Jerusalem, 1970).

267. The Nuremberg Laws on Citizenship and Race: September 15, 1935. http://frank.mtsu.edu/~baustin/nurmlaw2.html.

268. Israeli court rules Jews for Jesus cannot automatically be citizens. in *New York Times*, 1989.

269. Sand, S & Lotan, Y. *The Invention of the Jewish People*, xi, 332 p. (Verso, London; New York, 2009).

270. Halkin, H. Jews and their DNA. In *Commentary*, 2008.

271. Gorenberg, G. How do you prove you're a Jew? in *New York Times*, 2008.

272. Feldman, N. Orthodox paradox. In *New York Sunday Times Magazine*, 2007.

273. Sarna, JD. *American Judaism: A History*, xx, 490 p. (Yale University Press, New Haven, CT, 2004).

274. Lyall, S. Who is a Jew? Court ruling in Britain raises question. In *New York Times*, 2009.

275. Office of Management and Budget. Revisions to the standards for the classification of Federal data on race and ethnicity: Federal Register notice. 1997.

276. Jacobs, J. Are Jews Jews? Pop Sci Month 55:502–511, 1899.

277. Royal, CD, Novembre, J, Fullerton, SM, Goldstein, DB, Long, JC, Bamshad, MJ et al. Inferring genetic ancestry: opportunities, challenges, and implications. Am J Hum Genet 86:661–673, 2010.

INDEX

under Mourant, for Jewish
subgroups, 125–127
as population genetic markers,
123–124
serum banks for, 122
statistical analysis methods for,
131–132
transfusions between, 121
Bloom syndrome, 65–66, 74
Boas, Frans, 132
Bonne-Tamir, Batsheva, 47, 131,
137–138, 148
The Book of Destiny (Menton), 106
Book of Travels (Benjamin of Tudela), 112
Bradman, Neil, 87, 95, 96
BRCA genes, breast cancer and,
193–195
breast cancer, genetic research and
testing for, 192–195
BRCA mutations and, 193–195
Buerger, Leo, 50–51
Buerger disease, 50–52
ascertainment bias for, 51
Burne-Jones, Edward, 84
Burns, Edward, 145–146
Burt, Cyril, 158
criticism of, 159–160
Bustamante, Carlos, 141

Canavan disease, 64–65
cancer. *See* breast cancer, genetic research
and testing for; ovarian cancer,
genetic research and testing for
Cann, Rebecca, 107
Carmelli, Dorit, 131

Cavalli-Sforza, Luca, 88, 102, 148
blood grouping studies under,
127–132
dendritic trees and, development of,
129–131
education history of, 128
genetic distances and, development
of, 129
cephalic index, for Jewish groups,
10–11
A Certain People (Silberman), 205–206
Chase, Gary, 64
China, Jews in, 28
Christians
intermarriage with Jews, in Europe,
27–28
mental illness among, circa
1890–1902, 7
chromosomes
G6PD deficiency and, expression in,
41–48
Lyonization and, 44–45
in males, G6PD deficiency
expression, 42–43
in women, G6PD deficiency
expression, 44–45
Ciampa, Vicki, 144
Cilio, Roberta, 144
CMH. *See* Cohanim Modal Haplotype
coalescence theory
in CMH, 97–98
for Jewish genetic diseases, 70–72
mitochondria analysis and,
108–109
Cochran, Gregory, 161

R1 haplotype, in Y chromosome
analysis, 94–95
race
as conceptual term, xvi, 16–19
continental groups and, xvi–xvii
definition of, for humans, xvi–xvii,
17
environmental factors for, 17
ethnic groups and, xvi–xvii
genetic isolates and, xvii
genetic subgrouping and, through
evolution, 18–19
geographic origin and, 18
modern consensus on, 19
sociocultural factors for, 17–18
race science theory, during Nazi regime,
xv
red blood cells, G6PD deficiency and,
45
Reich, David, 108
Reinach, Theodore, 23–24
relaxification, with language, 103
religion, Jewish identity through,
199–200
through conversion, 216–217
in *National Jewish Population Survey of
2000–2001*, 199–200
religious conversion, Jewish identity
though, 216–217
research. *See* genetic research and testing
RH blood groups, 124–125
discovery of, 124–125
pregnancy and, with incompatible
parents discovery of, 124–125,
125

serum clumping reaction for, 124
Rhogam antibody, 125
Risch, Neil, 18, 165
Roden, Claudia, 169
Romanov, Alexis Nicolaievich, 64
Rosenberg, Noah, 135, 152
Rossetti, Dante Gabriel, 84
Rubinstein, Wendy, 193–194

Sachs, Bernard, 56
Sand, Shlomo, 210, 220
schizophrenia, among Ashkenazi Jews,
183–186
Scozzari, Rosario, 96
Seldin, Michael, 142
Sephardic Jews, 21
in *Genetic Disorders among Jewish People*,
54
intermarriage with Ashkenazi Jews,
xiv
in Jewish HapMap Project, 148–152
serum banks, for blood groups, 122
Shaltiel Gracian, Moshe, 106
Sheba, Chaim, 35–36
on disease susceptibility among Jews,
77–78
education history for, 37
favism and, study of, 38–39
malaria and, study of, 37–38
shiva, xvii
Shorto, Russell, 146
short-tandem repeats, in genomics,
134–139
Silberman, Charles, 205–206, 206
criticisms of, 206–207